LEUKEMIA

FROM DIAGNOSIS TO WINNING THE BATTLE

PERSPECTIVE • FAMILY • BLISS

*The story of being diagnosed with Leukemia
... and winning the battle.*

RYAN WOELFEL

Leukemia – From Diagnosis to Winning the Battle
Formatted and published by *Kouba Graphics, Inc., USA,* www.koubagraphics.com

Kouba
Graphics, Inc.

Printed in the United States of America

ISBN-13: 978-1-938577-05-5
ISBN-10: 1-938-57705-5

10   9   8   7   6   5   4   3   2   1

DEDICATION

This book is dedicated to Leukemia; my Wife; my Sister/ Donor; my Parents and In-laws; Medical Science; Transplant Physicians – Craig Rosenfeld (Medical City – Dallas), Brian Berryman (Medical City/Baylor – Dallas), Edward Agura (Medical City/Baylor – Dallas); Oncologists – Scott Stone (Medical Center of Plano); Infectious Disease Doctor, Howard Kussman (Medical Center of Plano); Internist – Jay Wallin (Mt. Carmel – Columbus, Ohio); Unplanned Teen Pregnancy/ Adoption; and most of all God for bringing all of these together.

SPECIAL ACKNOWLEDGMENTS AND THANKS

Would like to acknowledge the following individuals for their assistance with edits/suggestions for this book: Elisse Woelfel, my loving, supportive wife; My parents, Glenn and Patti Woelfel; My Sister/Donor, Lori Woelfel; Mora Kim, former colleague and friend of the family.

PAYING FORWARD

A percentage of all proceeds from the sale of this book will be donated to the Leukemia and Lymphoma Society.

CONTENTS

FOREWORD

BY BRIAN BERRYMAN

Ryan Woelfel is an incredible human being and has an extraordinary story to tell. As a member of his leukemia and transplant team, Ryan is my hero. His book, Leukemia – *From Diagnosis to Winning the Battle*, takes the reader on his journey of survival that no one should have to endure, especially a recently graduated 6½ year college student enjoying the time of his life with the love of his life. After reviewing his records, I was reminded of the medical facts of his leukemia diagnosis and chances for survival. Sometimes it is easier and less painful for me as a physician to keep to the impersonal statistics. The fact is Ryan Woelfel should not have survived. He did. I thank God and we are all better for it.

Ryan was diagnosed with Acute Myelogenous Leukemia (AML) while working on a new project in Columbus, Ohio on 11/14/2000. His white blood cell count was elevated 5-10 times above normal with circulating leukemic cells. He was severely anemic and his platelet count was so profoundly low that he was at risk for spontaneous life threatening bleeding. In typical form for Ryan, he debated whether to get himself checked at all. His symptoms were nonspecific, flu-like, as is often the case with leukemia. He was more concerned about his new position and his colleague. After his diagnosis of leukemia, he was worried more for his fiancée Elisse, his parents, his sister Lori, and his friends.

On 11/16/2000, Ryan underwent a bone marrow aspiration and biopsy back home in Dallas. It established the diagnosis of

Acute Myelogenous Leukemia. Medically, Ryan had several favorable prognostic features going for him: he was young, his performance status was excellent, he had no other major medical problems with no history of prior blood disorders. In addition, Ryan was truly blessed with an incredible support system of his parents, sister, friends and his future wife (and future attorney) Elisse. He had access to a great medical community here in Dallas. Ryan was and is intelligent and extremely determined to survive (stubborn, hard-headed some would say). Unfortunately, Ryan's bone marrow revealed complex acquired chromosomal abnormalities, so-called adverse risk disease. Statistically, it would be unlikely for Ryan to be cured with chemotherapy alone. For the best chance for a cure, Ryan would need an allogeneic (donor other than oneself) stem cell transplant.

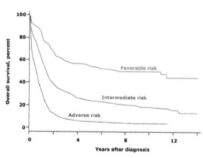

Data from Byrd, JC, et al. Pretreatment cytogenetic abnormalities are predictive of induction success, cumulative incidence of relapse, and overall survival in adult patients with de novo acute myeloid leukemia: Results from Cancer and Leukemia Group B (CALGB 8641). Blood 2002; 100:4325.

Ryan remarkably went into complete remission after his initial chemotherapy. Adverse risk AML often does not go into remission. His therapy was complicated by an invasive fungal infection which carries a mortality rate of 30-40%. Next, for a stem cell transplant, Ryan needed a donor. The best donor would be a full sibling but Ryan only had 1 sister to test, Lori. A sibling has a 25% chance of being a perfect match. Beyond his sister, a donor would have to be found in the registry which takes valuable time and risks relapse and the need for additional chemotherapy and their inherent toxicities. Fortunately, Lori was a complete match.

Ryan underwent an allogenic stem cell transplant (BMT) on 2/2/2001. He received the maximum humanly tolerated dose of radiation and chemotherapy to prepare his body. This regimen provided the most anti-leukemic benefit but had severe limiting organ toxicity. Severe liver toxicity can be associated with significant mortality rates of 80%. Again, Ryan survived and slowly recovered from the initial assault to his body only to face a life-long battle with chronic graft versus host disease (cGVHD) or rejection. From a leukemia standpoint, Ryan continues to be in complete remission, cured. He is 100% XX (female) – give him a hard time about that one.

I first met Ryan on 11/19/2002. He was dealing with chronic GVHD and secondary health issues. I was amazed by his medical story but more impressed by the young man's character and his accomplishments. Ryan is an honest, intelligent, compassionate and humble man. Because of his own medical experiences, Ryan felt the calling to pursue a medical career. This was amid his full-time job, new marriage, and the blessed additions to the Woelfel family, Landon and Huxton. Ryan joined our BMT team at Baylor in research and data collection. I was fortunate to work with him professionally for nearly a decade. Our program misses him dearly but knows the invaluable contributions he is making at UT Southwestern. (I will see you again, but not yet… not yet).

Ultimately, Ryan is living his best life possible. We should all learn this valuable lesson. He is a son to his amazing parents, a brother to his sister and life-saving donor Lori, a husband to the love of his life Elisse, and most importantly an amazing dad (Papa) to Landon and Huxton. For me, Ryan is my patient, colleague and friend. My hero.

CHAPTER 1:
NEW BEGINNINGS... AND INTERRUPTIONS

Life can often be unpredictable and full of uncertainty, which makes it fun, but can also make it terrifying at the same time. One seemingly normal day or moment could change the course of your life forever without you even noticing it's happening. It just so happens, my moment started with an instant message followed by a series of events where it would take years for me to understand the reason for all that was happening.

It all began, as most of my college stories did, with alcohol coupled with the addition of a computer and a group of friends that were actually more like brothers. Like most college guys, we were in the business of having copious amounts of fun with multiple members of the opposite sex. This was our focus most nights, which was reflected in my GPA, and that night in particular, when life hit me in the face with something I wasn't expecting or looking for – her name, Elisse.

After much alcohol consumption, my friends and I had stumbled upon a listing on the internet of all the college girls living near us who were also currently online. This was 1998, before "Tinder," "Match.com," "Call-me-Cupid," and all the other internet dating/hook-up sites that have now since exploded. This relatively new way of meeting girls seemed pretty easy and promising.

We decided to "instant message" a few of these girls (or IM for those of you who don't already know) and see how lucky we could get. The first one we IM'd was "mykie22" and the conversation was going quite well. "Mykie22" had wanted to meet up and gave us her phone number. At this point we were elated, as this was looking to be a pretty definite hookup for at least one of us, but we also figured she had to have roommates or friends who would also be willing to hook up.

My roommate, Chris, got on the phone and called her, but it was really more of a team effort as we all pitched in on what to say in order to avoid any periods of awkward silence. We were finding out this girl was not only willing and wanting to "hook-up" that night, but she also claimed to look like the "Noxzema Girl" (super-hot model at the time) and went by the name Sasha.

We had gotten her address and Chris, since he was the one who called her, took off to the shower and threw me the phone. I was now in charge with the phone in my hand, and was doing a stellar job of keeping the conversation going when out of nowhere, another friend, Dave, shouted out, "Hey Ryan, where did Chris go?" Normally this wouldn't have been an issue except Sasha thought she was talking to Chris and not me – busted!

Attempting to keep Sasha believing I was still the same guy she had been talking to all along proved difficult, as Sasha was no idiot. She immediately caught the mistake and said, "Wait a minute, I thought you were Chris." This was followed by many "ums" and "uhs" until I quickly came up with something I was sure would convince her I was Chris and he was I. I simply told her I was Chris Ryan, and my friend, Dave, calls me Ryan, but everyone else calls me Chris – "I go by both." I was sure this would work. It did not. Now I was really stammering, above and beyond um's and uh's. Sasha was definitely beginning to feel something was up and started to sound as if she was growing tired of this conversation quickly. I can't really recall what I said, but whatever it was, it worked and I was able to keep the conversation going.

What I had said not only salvaged the conversation, but it also must have caused Sasha to feel somewhat sorry for us, or what was about to happen to us, because after roughly 30 minutes or so, Sasha felt compelled to come clean and confess. Chris was about to be the butt of a glorious prank. Sasha went on to explain the elaborate scheme, and I of course became more and more intrigued and agreed it would be a great prank. She explained "mykie22" was a friend of hers who had just called her up telling her she just gave some random guys (us) her (Sasha's) phone number to call and wanted her to play along. The address we had been given was actually "mykie22's" neighbor, whom she was apparently not a huge fan of. The plan was to watch from their door as some guy – Chris – showed up and knocked on their neighbor's door acting like he was there to take part in the fun festivities they had (we had) discussed on the phone with the Noxzema look-alike. I thought this was a very well thought out plan and agreed to help ensure it would come to fruition.

Sasha and I continued to talk and I explained to her that since she now knew my name, it was only fair and customary that she tell me her real name. She said no, that she didn't give her name out to people she didn't know. I could be some crazy guy for all she knew. I indicated I was not, but that didn't sway her. I was not willing to take "no" for an answer, as we seemed to hit it off well, at least over the phone, and I wanted to see if this was worth pursuing. I had her number, thanks to "mykie22," but I didn't want to pursue if she had no interest. I figured if I could get her to give me her name, then that would be an indication she was interested. She continued to push back citing serial killers, rapist, etc., and she said let's leave it up to fate and told me to guess her name. I told her that was impossible as there are infinite possibilities. I asked her to give me a hint and she said it started with the letter "E." I said the first name that came to my mind and nailed it – can't argue with fate. She was absolutely shocked I got it, as was I. She proceeded to ask more questions to see if we had crossed paths at some point, as it didn't seem possible I would be able to just pull that name out of the air. I told her I just said the first name that came to mind and that was it. This of course resulted in a longer conversation, but we eventually got off the phone, as there was a prank that still needed to be done.

Right about the time we got off the phone, Chris returned ready to go, but was starting to have second thoughts. Great friend that I am, I encouraged him to follow-through, reminding him Sasha looked like the "Noxzema Girl," but the harder I pushed, the more suspicious he became, and he eventually backed out altogether.

I couldn't stop thinking of Elisse and how crazy all that was when about a week later, Dave got an instant message from none other than "mykie22." She and her friends, including Elisse, wanted to meet up somewhere. We picked a place we frequented for the free beer kegs and "all-you-can-eat" happy hour – Midnight Rodeo, or "Midnight Rope-A-Ho" as we frequently called it.

We told the girls what we would be wearing and told them to meet us at the cigarette machine. Our plan was full proof, as we didn't wear anything close to what we told them we would be wearing, and we sat in eye shot's view of the cigarette machine. This way if the girls were less than desirable, we'd count our blessings, move on, and never look back. There was just one problem with our plan – the girls had the same plan and needless to say, we never met.

A couple weeks went by and "mykie22" emailed us and invited us to a party at their apartment. When we showed up, the girls told us they were relieved we weren't the guys with the handlebar mustaches they had seen at the cigarette machine at our original meeting place. I was relieved Elisse was Elisse, as she was just as I had hoped she would be. This was evident from the look on my face in the picture we all took that night. She was by far the prettiest girl and frankly, I was dumbfounded as to what I possibly could've done right to be fortunate enough for her to be fully engaged in conversation with me at this time.

My life at that moment began to really take place. I felt an instant connection to Elisse. After getting home from the party, the first thing I did was call her and we spoke for hours on end. We made plans to get together the next day, as soon we would be breaking for Thanksgiving followed by finals and then Christmas. Although we were apart, physically, during this time, the phone kept us connected, and upon our return from the holidays, once we met up again, we never spent another day apart.

It was more than obvious to both of us fate had thrown us together in a most unique way. We both had older sisters who were the same age, mine named "Lori" and hers "Laura." We both had identical chin scars we had acquired as children. We were both in the college of communications, mine Telecommunications and hers Communication Studies. Additionally, neither of us were looking for a relationship or each other – it just kind of happened. Our inseparability was apparent to everyone and it would remain that way.

Four months into the relationship, my 23rd birthday was upon us and I brought Elisse home to meet my parents. What I had suspected from day one was confirmed. She got along with my family and friends with little to no effort; I knew she was the one. I couldn't imagine life without her and it wasn't long before we were talking marriage and kids and our future together. I remember it was Spring Break, March 1999, when she first told me she loved me and I had to ask her again to make sure I heard correctly. I remember her saying I was the first person she had no exceptions for. She made me feel like I was some prize, which floored me, because I always felt she was the prize that somehow, I had won. A few months later, we were engaged.

Graduation was now looming in the distance, and college life had come and gone. Texas Tech was just as fun as I had hoped it would be, if not more so, given the 6.5 years it took me to stretch a four-year Telecommunications degree into. Not having a class before 11:00 for most of my college career, taking two months off from attending some classes, and dropping half the classes in one semester only to retake them in another, will lead to this college tenure "stretching phenomenon."

I chose Texas Tech for two main reasons – the girl to guy ratio was 7:1 and it was ranked #2 in the nation for hottest girls and biggest party school. Needless to say, my focus in school was partying, meeting girls, and having fun. It wasn't until I met Elisse that I started getting more serious about school, graduating, and getting on with my life. In order to graduate with Elisse, I took 23 hours my last semester, and achieved what I thought would be sure to take me another year to complete – I had graduated and now had my whole life ahead of me. I guess it's true what they say about what motivates a man.

With graduation behind me, the next focus was landing a job. Most of this was worked out while in school, and I was in the final stages of interviewing, but this took some time, which gave us a chance to tour Europe as a graduation celebration. Though not apparent to us at the time, this month-long vacation proved valuable, as it provided us the opportunity to experience the best and worst of each other and really allowed us to gel together as a family, including my grandmother, sister and parents.

After returning from Europe, times were hectic as we were still planning a wedding, seeking employment, and getting used to settling in on our own. Even though I had already started the process of searching for employment as an undergrad, logistics still had to be worked out. All in all, from the time I first interviewed with Inet Technologies (an up and coming Telecom company) until I received the final word, took about six months. It was extremely nerve-racking to continue waiting on the official word to come through, and I was hearing from everybody, "...nothing's official until you sign on the dotted line...."

This constant barrage of unsolicited advice resulted in me constantly reassuring those concerned. In particular on one occasion, I had forwarded an email from the department director at Inet to my parents to keep them updated. To help ease my nerves, my mom replied by email reassuring me.

"Sweetie, don't worry so much. I'm sure they liked you and you wowed them – just be patient and it'll work out. Love Mom."

This was very reassuring, as mothers like to do for their sons, except that she had mistakenly hit "reply all" and that email went to not only me, but also the department's hiring manager, the director, and the HR representative at the company. I found this out when I received an email from the HR Rep. She wanted to know who this lady was and why she was calling me "sweetie." I was mortified. On the flip side though, I'm also pretty sure that email helped solidify the position for me as it, without a doubt, made me standout and left a memorable impression with the company.

Meanwhile, in great anticipation of landing the position, I had already moved to the Dallas area and began working as a subcontractor in the Telecom field while waiting for the position to come through. Elisse stayed with her parents in Conroe, working at a bank. We lived this way, only seeing each other on the weekends for most of the summer.

This living arrangement proved difficult in planning a wedding, as the wedding was set for Austin. We were planning on getting married in December, so we had time, but not a lot. We used our weekends together to meet with the various vendors for our wedding, which was difficult. In August, when my employment became official, things got a little easier and by the end of September, Elisse was hired as a Human Resources Coordinator for Amerimax Building Products in Dallas. With both of us now gainfully employed, we again began focusing more on our upcoming wedding and the beginning of our new lives together. This was the beginning of our new life…little did I know it was to be the beginning of another chapter that would threaten everything I held dear to me and the very life we were now beginning.

When we weren't busy working, planning the wedding, or hanging out with friends, we were caught up in the purchasing of our first home, which was a daunting, yet speedy task. It was a 3 bedroom, 2.5 bathroom house with wood floors, a study, a pool, and a fishpond – the perfect house for beginning a family. Our offer was accepted and we were on our way to making one of the biggest purchases of our lives. I'll admit we were a bit nervous to be making such a large purchase only three months out of college, but we were both employed and felt ready to take this next step.

Life was exciting and new at this point with everything slowly beginning to unfold for us. Work was going well, although, working in the real world took a little getting used to. Although I had worked a little through college, it was only part-time and I was not used to getting up and getting to work so early and getting back so late, but it was exciting to begin this new chapter.

On my first day at Inet, I found out I was slotted to go to Korea the next day; fortunately, however, our program director felt I needed to have more than just one day of training, before being sent out on my own, charged with supervising the installation and proper functioning of multimillion dollar equipment – so I was given two more days of training and then sent out. Although I was not sent to Korea, I was sent to Canada so I was quite a bit less nervous about the country, but just as nervous about the accountability and responsibility I was given. The trip went so well I soon realized the approximate 50% travel I was told I'd be doing actually translated to about 80%, as I was penciled in for upcoming trips to Alabama, Mississippi, Ohio, Georgia, New York, Chicago, Amsterdam, and, yes, Korea again. Fortunately, for some of the locations (New York 9/11), and unfortunately for others, I was only able to make about half of these trips, as something was beginning to happen to me that would not only change my direction and focus in life, but would shake me to the very core of my being and test everything I knew and thought I knew about myself.

Leukemic blasts – normal cells in my bone marrow that normally differentiate into various blood cells – only malignant, so unable to differentiate, but rapidly dividing; exponentially – were slowly beginning to take up home and space in my normal bone marrow. Although not apparent at the time, these leukemic blasts were beginning to overtake my bone marrow and halt the proper function of my bone marrow – production of cells which are crucial in fighting infection, carrying oxygen throughout the body, and clot formation. I wasn't even aware of the normal process, much less the malignant process that had begun to take place in me, and only in retrospect can I say about when these changes started to be noticeable.

On one of our many trips to Austin, planning for the wedding, Elisse and I were meeting with the photographer to take engagement photos. We were meeting in the hills of Austin – Cat Mountain – right around sunset to capture the right light and view and all was going as planned. While we were being positioned by the photographer, Elisse moved her hand in an upward direction inadvertently scratching me with her engagement ring. The insignificant scratch would not stop bleeding, and Elisse had to keep blotting my forehead with a tissue between shots. At the time, I thought nothing of it; however, Elisse did comment on how difficult it was to stop the scratch from bleeding. Little did we know at the time, it was because my platelets and the production thereof had been significantly decreased due to the malignancy growing inside my bone marrow.

We powered through the photo shoot, headed to meet my parents and friends for dinner, and then headed back up to Plano the next day. A couple of weeks went by, another trip down to Austin and back had come and gone, and I was prepping for yet another business trip – Ohio this time. That trip to Ohio was the most memorable trip I had ever taken and continues to hold that spot to this day and quite possibly will continue to do so for the rest of my life.

The morning of my trip, I remember turning on the TV to see if the election coverage had ended and if we had a new president, but to my amazement, along with the rest of the country, it still wasn't clear whether it would be Gore or Bush. In any case, my ride to the airport had arrived and I was on my way to Columbus. My co-worker and I landed in Columbus, got the rental car, and drove to the job-site to make sure all of our supplies arrived ahead of us and were pleased to see all was in order. We grabbed a quick bite to eat and retired to our rooms to get ready for the upcoming day.

I was feeling a bit sluggish after dinner and felt like I was beginning to come down with a cold or the flu. I debated as to whether or not to go to the doctor in the morning or just take some over-the-counter (OTC) meds and power through. I decided I would see how I felt the next morning and decide then. I called Elisse, who was addressing wedding invitations at the time, and told her I wasn't feeling too well and was off to bed early. We said goodnight and she said maybe I'll be able to come home a little early depending on how I felt and I agreed.

The next morning, sure enough, I felt worse and decided I would go to the doctor. I called the front desk and asked if there were any doctor offices close to our hotel and was told the closest one was about a half hour away, with the exception of Mt. Carmel Hospital, which was five minutes down the road.

I had the rental car, and knew if I didn't feel well and was unable to work, my co-worker would be stranded, so I left him a note saying I didn't feel well and was going to the doctor. I left the rental car keys and our job info at the front desk with the hotel staff and called a cab to go to Mt. Carmel.

When the cab dropped me off, I realized I was going to have to go through the ER, as everything else was still closed that early in the morning. I must admit, I felt pretty idiotic going to the ER for just a minor sore throat and flu like symptoms and this rang even more true when I gave the lady my insurance card and realized I was going to have to pay a $50 co-pay for this. I was beginning to seriously question how bad I was truly feeling and was starting to have second thoughts, but the cab had already left and I figured I was already there and decided to stay.

Soon I was called back to a large room with lots of people and rows of racks on the celling with curtains on them. I was asked the general questions about what my symptoms were, what kind of previous medical history I had, and how I was feeling. I mentioned my main complaint was my sore throat and my sluggishness, but had attributed that to all the back and forth Elisse and I had been doing between Dallas and Austin while planning our wedding, and didn't think too much of it. The nurse asked if there was anything else, and after thinking about it I mentioned a bruise on my leg still looking pretty nasty though two weeks had passed (another alcohol-induced injury). I also pointed out I had some white spots on the inside of my mouth that I had just noticed the night before. The nurse looked at the bruise and asked about some red spots on my forearm that looked like little claw marks. I attributed the spots to one of our cats. When the nurse asked me if there was anything else, I mentioned I had mono in high school and was wondering if the sluggishness, sore throat, and flu/cold like symptoms could all be just a reactivation of the mono virus. The nurse said possibly and drew some blood for some blood work.

About half the morning was now over and about 20 minutes later a doctor came to where I was and drew the curtain closed with a serious look on his face. I figured – crap – I do have mono again and now I'm going to have to call work and tell them I have to return home early. This was a huge deal to me, because this was my first real job out of college. I was working in the telecom industry, was able to name my salary, and now after only being employed with them for less than 3 months, I was going to have to pull out of this job leaving my co-worker high and dry, which was not the impression I wanted to give them.

How at the time I wished with all my heart, soul, and mind the doctor had said it was mono. But it wasn't. Suddenly, all my fears about work went out the window, as I was now being admitted to begin what would be the hardest fight of my life, and this would signal the very beginning of the end of everything I thought I knew about myself and my future.

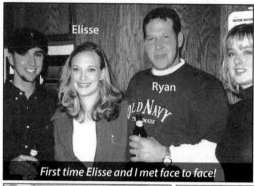

Elisse

Ryan

OLD NAVY

First time Elisse and I met face to face!

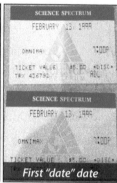

SCIENCE SPECTRUM

FEBRUARY 13, 1999

OMNIMAX   7:00P

TICKET VALUE $5.00   *DISC*
TRX 436790   ADU

SCIENCE SPECTRUM

FEBRUARY 13, 1999

OMNIMAX   7:00P

TICKET VALUE $5.00   *DISC*

First "date" date

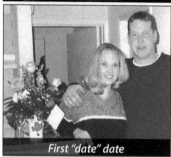

First "date" date

Ryan-
Before you leave for Austin

Remember to:
· Feed Freddy Fish
· make sure everything is locked up.
· Feed your fish w/ gold fish
· make sure the heater is on
  the lowest setting
· Remember that I LOVE YOU VERY much
· Be very careful + fasten your seat!
· Have a good time with your
  (soon to be my) Family!!!

I LOVE YOU NOW + Forever,

Elisse !!

IDEAL
Ideal Basic Industries
Cement Division

Sun, P.M.
10:30

Hi Honey
    Glad you got home
safely! We like you
to bring your friends
& it was a great visit!
— it just flew by. We
did like Elisse too,
but you do have
pretty good taste.
Take Care, study hard,
work hard, & if time
allows — play hard too!
We love ya bundles —US

First time Elisse met my parents

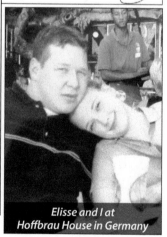

Elisse and I at
Hoffbrau House in Germany

Inet.

August 8, 2000

Ryan G. Woelfel
6780 State Highway, 29 West
Georgetown, TX 78628

Dear Ryan

Inet Technologies, Inc. and Tony Bailey are pleased to confirm the verbal offer extended to you at an annual salary of $45,800, payable semi-monthly, working in Inet's Program Management Department as an Installation Specialist. In addition, Inet will give you $1,500 to cover moving and relocation expenses, payable to you at the end of your first full pay period. Please note that if you decide to leave Inet within the first year of your employment, you will be required to reimburse the company for the relocation expenses.

Effective the first day of employment with Inet, you will be granted an option to purchase 100 shares of Inet's Common Stock under Inet's 1998 Stock Incentive Plan. The exercise price of your option will be the closing selling price of Inet's Common Stock on the date your option is approved. Your option will be exercisable for twenty-five percent (25%) of the option shares, upon your completion of each of the four (4) years of service with Inet, measured from the option grant date.

Inet is a high-growth, profitable enterprise that provides quality, innovative, competitively priced, state-of-the-art telecommunications products and support. Inet focuses on complete customer satisfaction and fosters an environment that encourages employee development. You will find your position to be both challenging and rewarding.

Keep in mind that all information pertaining to compensation is confidential. This offer is contingent upon acceptable results of your background check. If you have any questions about the offer or the company, please call Rachel Fulmer, Tony Bailey, or me.

Please sign the copy of this letter and return it in the enclosed envelope as formal acceptance of the offer within three working days from the date of this letter. We look forward to hearing from you by August 11, 2000. If you need more time to make your decision, please let us know.

Your interest in Inet is genuinely appreciated. We are confident that you will make a substantial contribution to our efforts and look forward to a favorable reply to our offer.

Sincerely,

Jim Oliphant

Jim Oliphant
Senior Vice President

Offer letter from Inet – first job out of college;
In the "real world" now

11-1-00

Dear Ryan and Elisse,
It was so good to see both of you at the party Saturday night.

Your mom told me about the two of you buying a new home, and Paw Paw and I are happy for you. Our only concern now is that you are adding more things to do before your wedding, but it will all work out for you I am sure. It will be an exciting time for you even though it will be busy.

Everything is "a go" on Margie's dress. I have had several people offer help with the appliques, so I feel it will work out the way you want it, and will be very

Post engagement party and two weeks prior to diagnosis

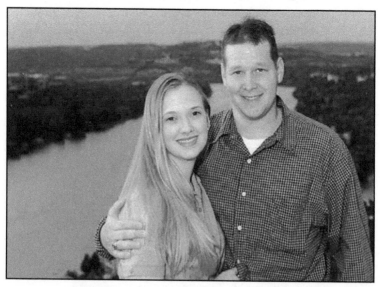

Engagement photos – you can barely see the scratch
that wouldn't stop bleeding, caused from Elisse's ring

Chapter 2: The Diagnosis

I wasn't quite fully processing what the doctor was saying when he told me most likely I had leukemia. This was because all I knew about leukemia at the time was it was a blood disease. Furthermore, he said I either had leukemia or a bone marrow virus and of course, I was clinging on the words, "bone marrow virus," as all I really had was a sore throat, so there was no way it could be leukemia – the big 'c' word. Also, I had always eaten plenty of green vegetables growing up, so I was protected from blood diseases – at least that's what my mom had always told me when she encouraged me to eat the healthy "stuff" – thanks Mom! It wasn't until the doctor told me, "I don't think you're quite understanding – leukemia kills, and that's even with treatment," that I began to grasp what was potentially happening to me. I asked the doctor how sure he was I had leukemia versus the bone marrow virus and he said based on preliminary results, he was about 80% sure I had leukemia. Of course though, I knew I had a bone marrow virus and would be out of the hospital as soon as the final tests came back.

As my denial was becoming more and more apparent, the doctor showed and explained to me what my blood work (complete blood count, CBC) showed. He said the cells that fight infection (white blood cells, WBC) in the normal population range from 4,500 to 11,000 and in my case they were 42,000, which could also signal I had a bad infection; however, even with an infection they were extremely elevated, more so than expected for just an infection. The protein responsible for carrying oxygen throughout the body (hemoglobin, HGB) in the normal population ranges from 12 to 15 and mine was 8.9, which explained my sluggish feeling. The cells responsible for clotting function (platelets, PLT) in the normal population range from 150,000 to 450,000, and mine were 11,000 (at 50,000, one can bleed to death from a cut while shaving). This explained the bruise on my leg and red spots on my arm, which I later found out were called petechiae – these spots I had attributed to our cats earlier. The final number that really drove things home was my blasts count. Blasts are normal in the bone marrow at 5% or less, as they are cells that haven't differentiated, or formed, into cells that serve a specific function. They reside and mature in the bone marrow and leak out once they become what they are genetically programmed to become. It's never normal to see blasts on blood work alone, because blasts never reside outside the bone marrow. This isn't the case, however, when the bone marrow becomes so packed full of blast cells. Once this occurs, blasts leak out and can be detected in blood work, as was evident in my case.

My CBC showed a blasts count of 62%, which translates to over half of the cells that comprised my blood were cells that could not fight infection, could not form clots, and could not carry oxygen throughout my body, because they were undifferentiated cells unable to mature to the next stage and perform the function for which they were destined to perform.

After convincing me how serious my condition was and how lucky it was I had decided to go to the doctor this morning, it was explained that I needed to be admitted to the hospital and given emergent platelet transfusions. Before being admitted for transfusions, and while I was still processing all I had just been told, I asked if I could make a few phone calls as I was on a business trip far from home. I needed to let my family know what was going on, so they could make arrangements as needed, as I wasn't sure how long I would be stuck in the hospital in Ohio. The doctor encouraged me to call my parents and let them know I was being admitted and he would see me in my room later to discuss a plan of care. With that, I began to try to wrap my head around who, and how I was going to call, and what I would possibly say to them.

My dad first came to mind, as I knew I could tell him and he would be able to hold it together, and I knew if I had told anyone else, they probably would have lost it, which in turn would have caused me to lose it. I remember thinking at the time that I didn't want to drop this on my dad while he was at work, but I didn't really have a choice. I knew I couldn't and wouldn't be able to tell my mom, and I was planning on telling Elisse later after I spoke with the doctor again and had more information.

Calling my Dad was by far the hardest thing I had to do up to that point, but it was a very "matter of fact" phone call. I basically said I hadn't been feeling well, so I went to the doctor and when they did blood work, they said it looked like I could have leukemia, but also possibly a bone marrow virus, which is what I was still thinking I had. He asked if leukemia was a type of cancer and I told him I wasn't sure, but the doctor would be seeing me later in the day and I was being admitted for observation and platelet transfusions for the time being. He asked if I felt sick and how I was doing and I told him I didn't really feel sick and that's why I was sure it was a bone marrow virus and not leukemia. I told him there was no way I could tell Mom and for him to wait to tell her until he saw her that night, so he wouldn't ruin her day. We said our goodbyes and I told him

I'd call them tonight to give them an update after I spoke with the doctor again.

Once I got to my hospital room, I had to call my office and let them know what was going on. I called my manager back home and told him I had basically been admitted to the hospital for observation. I explained my blood work came back a little off, and I wasn't sure how long I would be off the job site, but would update them as I got more information. My manager said not to worry about contacting my co-worker traveling with me and just take care of myself and keep them updated. This was a relief, as I had only been working there for just under 3 months. The rest of the day basically entailed me sitting in the hospital bed getting platelet transfusions with a thousand thoughts running through my mind while waiting on the doctor. Thoughts like – Is this really happening? Am I really that sick? How and what am I going to tell Elisse? What's she going to say or do? When's the doctor coming? When am I getting out of here? How is my family going to take it? What about our house? – and on and on and on.

Just as I was beginning to go crazy, a knock came at the door and the doctor I had talked to in the morning walked in and said, "Well I was wrong." Immediately I thought – "Hell ya!" I knew I didn't have leukemia, and it was just a mix up – but before I could say anything, the doctor continued, "I'm now 100% sure you have leukemia rather than a bone marrow virus and we're going to have an oncologist speak with you shortly." This was the news I had been dreading all day and now it was time to let Elisse know, but then the oncologist walked in.

He mentioned he knew it was a tough, almost impossible thing to hear, but he wanted to be upfront and to the point.

I asked him what the next step was and he said in order to confirm the diagnosis, even though he was 100% sure at this point, I would have to undergo a bone marrow biopsy. He explained this is when a large needle is pushed into the lower hip and through the bone into the marrow and then the marrow is drawn back up into the needle, along with a piece of the bone. These samples are then viewed under a microscope to get a more concrete exact confirmatory diagnosis. He mentioned this was not a pleasant procedure in the least bit and being that I was in Ohio on business, with no family here, I would most likely want to be treated at home. He indicated a bone marrow biopsy is the only way to get a confirmatory diagnosis, but it would be pointless doing a bone marrow biopsy while in Ohio, because, as soon as I got back home and checked in to a local hospital, they'd be repeating it.

The best plan of care at this point was to give me enough PLT transfusions to get my PLT count up from 11,000 to 50,000. The oncologist explained with my PLT count currently being at 11,000, something as insignificant as bumping my hand on a chair could cause me to bleed to death, so PLT transfusions were crucial at this point. As soon as they reached 50,000, it would be safe enough for me to get on a plane; although, I still needed to be extremely careful.

As soon as I landed, I was to check into the hospital nearest to my home and tell them I had just been diagnosed with leukemia while on a business trip and I urgently needed to be admitted immediately to begin chemotherapy. Once I wrapped my head around this and processed what I could, I knew I couldn't put it off any longer. It was time to make the call that would prove to be the hardest one to make – calling Elisse.

Eventually, I was able to muster up enough strength to begin dialing after hours of procrastination. I knew she was all alone, and I had no barometer with which to measure how she would take this. We had never been faced with such a scary scenario since becoming a couple, and no one is really ever prepared to hear what I was about to tell her.

She answered the phone and the first thing I said to her was, "Well, I'm coming home early" and she was very happy to hear that. I was just about to tell her why, when she asked me if there was any way I could call her right back – Frasier was on TV and she was in the middle of addressing wedding invitations. Now this was an important time in the "world of Frasier," as everyone was wondering if Daphne and Niles would or wouldn't hook up, so I understood the importance and told her no problem, and would call her back after it was over. This also gave me some more time to wrap my head around what I was going to say.

Frasier was on the TV in my hospital room as well, so I could see when it was over and with the credits rolling, I called Elisse. When she picked up the phone, she said, "So you're coming home early? That's good. Did you finish early?" I told her I was coming home early for another reason and that I was in the hospital. She asked if I got electrocuted or something – she knew what I was doing required powering down large computer systems and powering them back up. This of course didn't show too much confidence in her thinking I knew what I was doing, but when I told her the reason I was coming home, there was nothing but dead silence. This silence was broken by my re-assuring her something must be mixed up and when I get home it'll all get sorted out. What I didn't know at the time was when Elisse was a child, their next door neighbors lost their daughter to leukemia, so it really hit home for her. Telling her this, miles away, was excruciating – she was all by herself and there was nothing that could be done but anxiously wait.

As a new patient being thrown into this new journey, although I didn't have a firm diagnosis, my concern for her was far more than any concern I felt for myself. I think this is a recurring theme with most patients dealing with a diagnosis of cancer. As the patient, we can deal with the information we're given because we are the ones with the cancer and receiving the treatment. The family of a cancer patient is often left feeling helpless, because they feel there's nothing they can do. I can assure you without a doubt, Elisse was my sole focus of getting through this diagnosis and she helped me through more than she could ever possibly know.

As the night went on, after 8 units of PLT transfusions throughout most of the night and into the early morning of the next day, my PLT count reached 57,000 and I was discharged with instructions to go straight to the airport, land, and go straight to the hospital. I called for a cab, got to the airport and flew out on the red eye. Elisse met me in Dallas and we were on our way, but before checking into the hospital, I wanted to stop by the apartment first. I was exhausted and just wanted to rest a bit. I walked into the apartment, walked right to the phone and called the hospital, as instructed, saying I had just been diagnosed with leukemia and I needed to be admitted. I soon found out the complexities of insurance. I couldn't just walk into the hospital to be admitted under the care of an oncologist. I first needed a referral from my primary care physician, PCP.

As soon as I got off the phone with the hospital, we took off to get a referral from my PCP whom I had seen earlier for recurrent nose bleeds. We calmly walked in and explained the situation and urgency with which I needed to be seen and the triage nurse looked up at us with a blank expression on her face and said, "Looks like we can get you in sometime in the afternoon," to which Elisse, not so calmly, asked if she had just heard anything we had just said. She then proceeded to just about jump over the counter when the nurse finally started to realize, as did everyone else in the waiting area, just how serious this was and we weren't leaving until we were seen, or at the very least, had our referral.

At that moment, miraculously, the customer service we experienced greatly improved. In fact, within a few minutes we had our referral and it was faxed to the hospital, and we were on our way back to our apartment. We walked in and called the hospital and they said everything was set up and we needed to come to the hospital around 4PM to be admitted and I would see the oncologist around 6PM that night.

Now that we had a little bit of time before having to be up at the hospital, there was something we still had to take care of in the midst of everything else. Remember the house we were slotted to close on? Well, we had to go to the title company to hand them our down payment, complete the closing process, and get the keys to our first home. This was a huge leap of faith, as neither of us knew what was going to happen in the upcoming months. Perhaps if we had canceled the closing of the house, it would have seemed like an admission that something was wrong with me. Denial is a pretty powerful thing when you're told you are sick and quite possibly could die when you're only 24 and feel like you have your whole future ahead of you.

I'll never forget the look on the faces of the people at the title company when we handed them our check and Elisse's eyes were welling up with tears. They could tell something was terribly wrong as they handed us the keys to our new home. It was obvious Elisse's tears weren't from joy.

As we pulled up to our new home, the first thing we did was check the mail and there was a letter in the mailbox that was glaring at me. It was a thank you note from the Leukemia and Lymphoma Society for a donation we made at one of their fundraising events months earlier. "Have a Nice Day Café" was hosting an event that charged $20 at the door. The cover got you all you could eat and drink for three hours – the main reason I had gone that evening. While in line, I joked about the wait and cost because I didn't know anyone with leukemia or lymphoma, and didn't see how it would ever benefit me. Words cannot describe what or how I felt as I opened that letter from the Leukemia and Lymphoma Society thanking me for my donation that would help support research for the very disease I had just been diagnosed with. The irony would definitely fit well in an Alanis Morrissett song.

Later, when we arrived at the hospital, after getting through the admittance process, we were shown to my room – our new home. I say "our" because Elisse was right there with me, never leaving my side throughout my hospitalization, and this, too, would be a recurring event throughout this journey.

Soon, after our arrival, it was apparent luck was on my side, as my first oncologist, Dr. Scott Stone walked in – a fellow former Tech student as well. He entered the room and addressed Elisse and I as "the peas," since we were both crammed in the twin hospital bed together side by side. We got right to it. He told me from what the medical records he had received from my previous night's stay in Columbus showed, he too was sure

I had leukemia. He went on to explain we needed to see how aggressive and what subtype of leukemia I had before we could really discuss treatment options and a plan of care. This would require a bone marrow biopsy. He explained the procedure, which sounded just as frightening as it did when it was explained to me the night before with the doctors I saw in Ohio. He said to try to get some rest and the biopsy would be done first thing in the morning. I learned that night getting rest in a hospital is impossible and this lesson would remain true throughout all my hospitalizations.

Morning came with a knock on the door and the doctor walking in with his "biopsy kit." We made some small talk – joked about how getting rest in a hospital is a well-known joke amongst hospital folk, and then it was time. Elisse got out of the bed and stood next to my side giving her hand to squeeze. The doctor began by giving some local anesthetic, lidocaine, through a needle and then began depressing the biopsy needle into my hip as I lay face down. I can only describe the biopsy procedure as feeling a great deal of pressure in the lower back, with a sudden forward lunge, which occurs when the bone breaks under the needle. The next thing that occurs is the drawing up, or "aspiration" of the bone marrow, which feels like a cross between a bee sting and an electric shock that is constant and inward radiating outward. Once the marrow has been aspirated into the needle along with the piece of bone, the needle is pulled out very slowly, as it tends to grab on the bone as it backs out causing a bit of upward thrust as the needle exits the biopsy site – not a pleasant procedure, but necessary nonetheless. When Dr. Stone finished, he applied pressure to the site, as a bandage was wrapped around me and said he would return when the results were back for review in a few hours. In the meantime, an IV was started and fluids were administered, which was preparing me for the next step – treatment.

After a few hours and lots of fluid, the doctor came back and explained to me based on what he saw under the microscope, as expected, I did in fact have leukemia. This was the confirmation I had been dreading, as this was confirmatory proof. My bone marrow – responsible for making all of the blood cells necessary for life and the basis of the immune system – was full – approximately 100% of cells stuck in their undifferentiated blast state. These cells, since they were immature and unable to mature, were functionless, except in the profound function they were only able to perform in, excel in – filling my marrow, via their rapidly dividing capabilities and crowding out the needed functional cells necessary for life. In effect, they were silently killing me. This is the reason I had so many blasts showing up in my blood work the night before. They were leaking out of my marrow because my marrow was full of them. This also explained why my PLT and other counts were so low, as they weren't being produced any more by my malignant bone marrow.

As Dr. Stone was explaining this to Elisse and me, a whirlwind of thoughts came rising up. Is this really happening? How can this be for real? The only thing that's wrong with me is my sore throat. I remember explaining to Dr. Stone that I felt totally fine and didn't understand how I could feel this well if this were in fact happening. He calmly said I may feel well, but clearly, I am not well based on everything my body is saying via the pathology reports from the bone marrow biopsy and the blood work. Now with the diagnosis confirmed and now beginning to sink in, we started to talk about a plan of care.

It was November 17, 2000, and Elisse and I were 29 days from being married. We had just closed on a house, and now we listened as the doctor told us my mortality and morbidity percentages based on the type of cancer I had. I had acute leukemia of the myeloid lineage (blood line) – commonly referred to as acute myeloid leukemia (AML), and the subtype I had was M4 – myelomonocytic leukemia. This meant that in the blood lineage, as cells differentiate from myeloblast – blast in the myeloid (blood) line, to normal blood cells, my cells were arrested at this myelomonocytic stage and would not/could not develop any further.

At this stage, all we knew for sure is that I would undergo chemotherapy – commonly referred to as "7+3," or Idarubicin and Ara-C. This chemotherapy was called induction chemo, because its job was to eradicate the cancer from my bone marrow and "induce" remission. As Dr. Stone explained what would happen over the course of the next few weeks, we were learning new terms like "neutropenia," "neutrophils," "ANC" (absolute neutrophil count), "neutropenic fever," "nadir," "count recovery," and the one term we held onto most – "remission."

Dr. Stone also told us it was unlikely I would be out of the hospital in time for our wedding, and if I was, I certainly wouldn't feel up to it, so he said it was best to postpone it for now and reassess once I was out of the hospital, should everything go well. We had been planning our wedding for almost a year. Twelve of our friends were planning to be in our wedding party and there were about 300 people who were invited guests. Elisse and our mothers had the daunting tasks of making the phone calls to let everyone know the wedding was being indefinitely postponed. We were slotted to begin chemo the next day.

One thing Elisse and I weren't thinking of at this time was something our mothers and the nurses definitely were – my sperm, or lack thereof once I was through with chemo. The same day, although all at different times, the near certainty of my sterility was brought up along with the question of whether or not we had discussed sperm banking. Of course, neither of us had thought of this, as Elisse and I were still processing and absorbing my cancer diagnosis and everything it entailed. Our whole lives had been turned upside down, with all of our future plans hanging in limbo, and this had all occurred within the past couple days. We knew we wanted kids in the future, so it was an easy decision and the next step was to work out the logistics of how this would occur given the need for me to begin chemotherapy as soon as possible. Luckily the hospital we were at had a facility set up just for this purpose and it was a seamless process for us to begin prior to the initiation of chemo. Due to the scheduling of chemo, I was able to make one deposit before and one deposit after, but within the 48-hour safe zone of chemo, when the sperm would still not be affected by it.

Although still quite apprehensive about the uncertainties that lie ahead, I was ready to get going as I didn't really have a choice if I wanted to get on with my life and all it had to offer. After the nurses left and my parents left, it was just Elisse and I left in the room to try to process what we had learned over the past couple of days and what it meant for our future.

Tomorrow was fast approaching and it was a big day – it would be the start of my treatment regimen which consisted of seven days of continuous chemotherapy with one drug, along with three days of another drug. These drugs had the potential to put me in remission, make me more sick, or result in multi-organ failure, eventually resulting in death. I was hoping for the first option of remission, though fully aware "all of the above" were all definite potential outcomes. With that the lights were shut off – sleep somehow came.

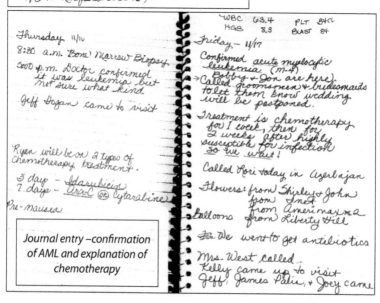

Wednesday 11/15
about 6:30 p.m. admitted to Medical Center of Plano

Redid blood work and confirmed way abnormal

WBC 57.2 (white blood count

HGB 8.4 (red blood count)

PLT 50 CL (platelet count)

BLASTs 42

6 x (2 pints blood)   12
10 x (platelets)   100

Admission to Hospital for chemo after returning home from Columbus, OH the night before

Thursday 11/16
8:30 a.m. Bone Marrow Biopsy
5:00 p.m. Doctor confirmed it was leukemia but not sure what kind.
Jeff Hogan came to visit

Ryan will be on 2 types of chemotherapy treatment.

3 day – Idarubicin
7 day – AraC or Cytarabine
Pre-nausea

Journal entry – confirmation of AML and explanation of chemotherapy

WBC 63.4   PLT 84 CL
HGB 8.3   BLAST 84

Friday – 11/17
Confirmed acute myelocytic leukemia (m-4)
Called groomsmen & bridesmaids to let them know wedding will be postponed.

Treatment is chemotherapy for 1 week, then for 2 weeks after highly susceptible for infection so we wait!

Called Lori today in Azerbajan

Flowers: from Shirley & John
   from Inez
Balloons from Amerimax x 2
   from Liberty Hill

We went to get antibiotics

Mrs. West called.
Kelly came up to visit
Jeff, James Palu, & Joey came

```
RUN DATE: 11/17/00                          MEDICAL CENTER OF PLANO LAB
RUN TIME: 2000                                    3901 W 15TH ST
                                              PLANO, TX  75075-7738


                                              CUMULATIVE REPORT


Patient: WOELFEL,RYAN G                              (Continued)
***************************************************** * * * H E M A T O L O G Y * * * **
                                            ---- COMPLETE BLOOD COUNT ----

Day                                          3          1
Date                                      11/17/00   11/15/00
Time                Reference Units          0654       2030

WBC                 (4.0-10.5) K/mm3       63.4(A)CH  57.2(B)CH

      (A)  Called by:  PB to GINA 11/17/00 0810
      (B)  Called by:  MMG to NANCY 11/15/00 2122

CORRECTED WBC                K/mm3          63.4        57.2
RBC                 (4.7-6.0) M/mm3         2.31 L      2.35 L
HGB                 (13.5-18.0) gm/dl       8.3 L       8.4 L
HCT                 (42.0-52.0) %           23.0CL     23.5(C)CL

      (C)  Called by:  MMG to NANCY 11/15/00 2123

MCV                 (78.0-100.0) UM3        99.6       100.3 H
MCH                 (27.0-31.0) MCMCGM      35.7 H      36.0 H
MCHC                (32.0-36.0) %           35.9        35.9
RDW                 (11.5-14.0)             17.5 H      17.4 H
PLT                 (150-450) K/mm3         34CL        50 L
MPV                 (6.0-9.5) fl            7.1         7.8
SEGS                (32-57) %               1 L         3 L
LYMPH               (25-33) %               7 L         29
MONOCYTE            (0-10) %                8           5
BLAST               (0-0) %                 84 H        42 H
IMMATURE CELL               %                           21
DIFF COMMENT                                            PATH REV
HYPOCHROMIA         (NEG)                               1+
POIKILOCYTOSIS      (NEG)                               1+
ANISOCYTOSIS        (NEG)                   1+          1+
SMUDGE CELLS                %                           6
PLT ESTIMATE                               DECREAS     NORMAL

***************************************************** * * * S E R O L O G Y * * * ****

Day                                          2          1
Date                                      11/16/00   11/15/00
Time                Reference Units          0850       2030

CMV IGG             (<0.91) ISR                        0.22(D)

      (D)  CMV IgG Antibody Result Interpretation:
                          < 0.91 ISR:  Negative
                    0.91 - 1.09 ISR:  Equivocal
                          > 1.09 ISR:  Positive
```

Lab work from admission day and day prior to initiation of chemo.
Blasts doubled from 42% to 84% in two days. Normal would be no blasts

THE UNIVERSITY OF TEXAS
SOUTHWESTERN MEDICAL CENTER
AT DALLAS

Cytogenetics Laboratory
Southwestern Pathology Consultative Services

Department of Pathology
5323 Harry Hines Blvd./Dallas, Texas 75390-9073
Telephone: (214) 648-3782 Fax (214) 648-5646

Patient: Ryan WOEFEL

Hospital No.: Medical Center of Plano #966541192

Physician: Stone, S.

Date Received: 11-16-2000

Specimen: Bone marrow

Reason: Acute myeloid leukemia

Lab No.: M00-2960

D.O.B./Age: 2-26-1976

Date of Report: 11-22-2000

Number of Cells Counted:	15	
Modal Chromosome Count:	46	
Number of Cells Analyzed:	15	
Number of Cells Karyotyped:	2	

Level of Band Resolution: <400

Banding Method: GTW

Karyotype: 46,XY,del(7)(q36),del(16)(q13q22),t(16;18)(p11.2;p11.32) [14 cells]/46,XY [1 cell]

Impression: Male with an abnormal clone and cytogenetically normal cell(s) in bone marrow

COMMENTS:
   Dividing cells from overnight and 48-hour cultures of this specimen were examined. Deletion in the long arm of chromosome #16 is a recurring cytogenetic abnormality in acute myeloid leukemia (AML), which is distinguished clinically from inversion of chromosome #16 by its lack of association with a good prognosis (ref. 1). Deletion in the long arm of a #7 chromosome is also a recurring aberration in AML; it was associated with an intermediate prognosis in a large recently reported study (ref. 2).
   Preliminary results (46,XY,7q-,-16,18p+,+mar [8 cells]/46,XY [1 cell]) were telephoned to Gennie Howe in Dr. Stone's office on 11-20-00.

References:
   1. Marlton P, et al. Cytogenetic and clinical correlates in AML patients with abnormalities of chromosome 16. Leukemia 1995;9:965-971.
   2. Grimwade D, et al. The importance of diagnostic cytogenetics on outcome in AML: Analysis of 1,612 patients entered into the MRC AML 10 trial. Blood 1998;92:2822-2338.

Nancy R. Schneider, M.D.

Nancy R. Schneider, M.D., Ph.D., Co-Director, Cytogenetics Laboratory
Frederick F. B. Elder, Ph.D., Co-Director, Cytogenetics Laboratory
Kathleen S. Wilson, M.D., Associate Director, Cytogenetics Laboratory

*Cytogenetics Report (chromosomal analysis) –
In my case, part of chromosome 16 broke and fused with a part of
chromosome 18 that broke apart. Together these abnormalities
demonstrated a poor prognosis and a high probability of relapse.*

```
Acct #: E00966541192                    Location: E.4W        E.405-A
DOB: 02/26/76   24/M                    Status: ADM IN
Unit #: E000518027
                                        Procedure Date: 11/16/00
Specimen: PL:800-9075                   Received Date : 11/16/00
                                        Physician: Stone,Scott A M.D.
```

TISSUES:

　　　BONE MARROW, NOS - ASPIRATE AND BIOPSY

CLINICAL HISTORY:
Acute myelogenous leukemia

GROSS DESCRIPTION:

　　　　　　　　　　　　BONE MARROW REVIEW

WBC	57.2	HCT	23.5	MCHC	35.9
RBC	2.35	MCV	100.3	PLTS	50,000
HGB	8.4	MCH	36.0	RDW	17.4

The specimen is received in Pen-Fix, labeled "BM core", and consists of a 1.0cm long, firm, brown cylindrical core of bone marrow which averages 0.2cm in diameter. The entire specimen is submitted after decalcification.

Also received in Pen-Fix, labeled "BM clot", is a 1.2x1.0x0.2cm, soft red-brown irregular portion of blood clot. The entire specimen is submitted. (2)

Also received is a peripheral blood smear labeled with the patient's name and a complete blood count indices sheet labeled with the patient's name.

　　Dictated by: MILONOVICH,SHEILA P
　　Entered: 11/17/00 - 1351 E.LAB.JS

MICROSCOPIC DIAGNOSIS:
The peripheral blood smear shows the white cell count is elevated. The vast majority of circulating white blood cells represent blasts. These cells average 16-20 micrometers in greatest diameter. The nuclear to cytoplasmic ratio is very high. The chromatin fabric is relatively fine and some cells have multiple small visible nucleoli. The cytoplasm to the blasts is smooth and relatively clear. A few vacuoles are identified. No distinct granules or Auer rods are identified. A much smaller subpopulation of circulating white blood cells represent monocytes, lymphocytes and rare granulocytic forms. Occasional nucleated red blood cells are also present. The platelet count does appear reduced in number. The red blood cell morphology is relatively normochromic and normocytic. The slide aspirate smear preparations are markedly cellular. The vast majority of nucleated cells represent relatively primitive appearing blast type cells. The cells have similar cytomorphic features to those previously described. The rare cells appear to contain a few intracytoplasmic azurophilic granules. Scattered small numbers of eosinophils are also identified. The bone marrow core biopsy consists of a single intact needle shaped fragment of medullary bone. The cellularity is virtually 100%. The vast majority of nucleated cells represent primitive blast-type cells. The cytomorphology is similar to those previously described. There does appear to be scattered eosinophilic cells in the background. The clot section contains numerous hematopoietic particles entrapped in blood clot. The particles show virtually 100%

```
SPEC #: PL:800-9075        PATIENT: WOELFEL,RYAN G        #E00966941192   (Continued)
```

```
Specimen: PL:800-9075        Received: 11/16/00-1116        (Continued)
```

MICROSCOPIC DIAGNOSIS: (Continued)
cellularity. The vast majority of nucleated cells represent primitive blast-type cells. Special stain for iron shows adequate stainable iron store deposition best identified on slide aspirate smear preparation.

FINAL DIAGNOSIS

　　PERIPHERAL BLOOD SMEAR, BONE MARROW ASPIRATION AND CORE BIOPSY):
　　　ACUTE MYELOGENOUS LEUKEMIA; SEE COMMENT

　　Dictated by: ALDRED,KEITH MD
　　Entered: 11/17/00 - 1408 E.LAB.JS

PATHOLOGIST COMMENTS:
Flow cytometry performed on this biopsy material shows the immunophenotypic characteristics of acute myelogenous leukemia (non-promyelocytic). The cytomorphology of the blasts and immunophenotypic markings are highly suggestive of at least a component of the blast cells with a monocytic lineage. Appropriate clinical correlation and follow-up are recommended.

Diagnostic Confirmation of Acute Myelogenous Leukemia
(AML) based on morphology (how my specimen looked under the microscope)

Dec 9. 2004. 12 41PM   INTGHL FLOW

Cellular Immunology Laboratory
University of Texas Southwestern Medical Center
Parkland Health & Hospital System
6000 Harry Hines Blvd, NB6. 126
Dallas, TX 75390-9072   Phone: (214) 648-4078
Fax: (214) 648-4091

Name: **Woefe, Dan**   214

PSL #: **11808**   Age: **24 Years**

Sex: **M**   Race: **UN**

CLINICAL INFORMATION
Sample: **Bone Marrow**

Sample Date: **11/16/2000**   Report Date: **11/20/2000**

Referral Doctor: **Stone**

Other Doctor: **Keith Aldred, MD**

Referral Institution: **Medical City - Dallas**

Referral ID#: **966541192**

Secondary Referral:

Clinical History: **Evaluate for AML.**

Previous Cases: **None**

LEUKOCYTE MARKER PANEL PERFORMED: Acute Leukemia - Adult

CD34/CD14/CD45/CD38	CD36/CD64/CD45/CD34	CD10/CD22/CD20/CD34
m.Kappa/m.Lambda/CD20/CD19	CD8/CD5/CD3/CD4	CD16/CD56/CD45/CD11b
CD7/CD13/HLA-DR/CD34	CD61/CD2/CD45/CD34	CD15/CD33/CD34/CD11b
MPO/icCD79a/CD45/CD34	TdT/icCD22/icCD3/CD33	

MORPHOLOGY:
The cytospin and smear preparations reveals a predominant population of medium to large blasts characterized by ovoid to indented or convoluted nuclear contours, immature chromatin pattern with multiple nucleoli, moderately abundant basophilic cytoplasm with occasional small azurophilic granules. No Auer rods are seen. Scattered background haematopoietic elements are also identified including eosinophils, some with mixed basophilic and eosinophilic granules, dysplastic erythroid and granulocytic elements.

IMMUNOPHENOTYPIC FINDINGS:
Immunophenotypic analysis reveals a 75-86% population of medium to large-sized (forward light scatter properties) myeloblasts with the following immunophenotype: CD45(moderate +), CD34(partial +), CD38(+), CD33(partial dim +), CD13(predominantly +), CD11b(partial dim +), CD15(partial +), CD14(-), CD16(-), CD36(partial +), CD64(partial +), CD4(partial +), CD2(partial +), CD7(dim +), HLA-DR(+), TdT(-), MPO(+), other lymphoid and myeloid antigens(-). Also identified are: 3.8% maturing granulocytic elements with decreased orthogonal light scatter properties (indicative of hypogranularity), 10.8% monocytes, 0.23% erythroid elements, 3.3% small (forward light scatter properties) mature, T lymphocytes (CD4:CD8 = 1.4:1), 0.76% NK cells, 0.05% maturing B-lineage precursors (hematogones), 1.5% small, mature, polytypic B lymphocytes (kappa:lambda = 1.2:1) and 0.02% plasma cells.

INTERPRETATION:
The findings indicate an acute myeloid leukemia, non-promyelocytic, with immunophenotypic evidence of monocytic differentiation. Final interpretation requires morphologic, cytogenetic and clinical correlation.

Results called to Dr. Keith Aldred (voicemail) on 11/17/00 by MJL, MD.

RESIDENT/FELLOW: PATHOLOGIST: _____
M. Jane Latimer, MD

Medical City - Dallas
7777 Forest Lane
Building A-12 South
Dallas, TX 75230
ATTN: Dept. of Pathology

Phone: 972/566-7105
Fax: 972/566-7165

Printed: 11/20/2000 @ 10:14:18 AM

*Diagnostic Confirmation of Acute Myelogenous Leukemia
(AML) based on morphology (how my specimen looked
under the microscope)*

34

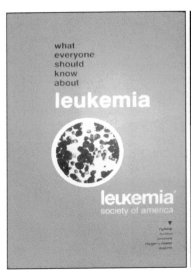

Book given to me
on what leukemia was –
patient education

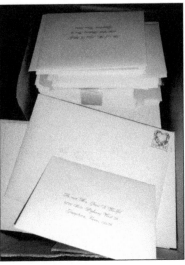

Wedding invitations Elisse
was addressing when I
contacted her to inform her of me
possibly having leukemia

Dec.17

Dearest Elisse,
We got word last night about
Ryan's leukemia and had a very
rough time sleeping while thinking
of you all and the shock and grief
you must be going through.
Please know that you are in our
prayers - as well as being on our
church's prayer list and about a
half dozen others around town.
May our Lord wrap His loving arms

First news getting out that I had been diagnosed with cancer

I'm enclosing photos from the party in the hopes that you can smile a bit while looking at them.

Today is Margi's Thanksgiving Feast at school so I made cranberry jello jigglers in the shape of leaves and acorns. I didn't think they would eat cranberries so I improvised.

If you have the strength, please give your folks and Elissa a big hug and imagine one from us.

God bless and keep you in His loving arms.

Love,

Kim, Mark, Margi, and Elissa

December 17

Wishing you a *speedy* recovery!

Dearest Ryan,

We just got word last night about your condition and are trying to recover from the shock – as, I'm sure, are you! Please know, and take to heart, that you are in our prayers, as well as those of our church and a good half-dozen other churches around town! Prayer warriors unite!

Supportive card – half dozen churches around San Antonio were praying for me

Dear Elissa,

I was so sorry too hear about Ryan. I wish there was something I could do or say, but I know there isn't.

Keep on praying Elissa and I will be praying with you. May God Bless the both of you and hold you close, till you both feel his Love, surrounding you, and never let you go, I hope your holidays will be full of joy and Love. I'll pray for you both.

Love Your friend
Nelson & Martha

CHAPTER 3: CHEMO (INDUCTION)

With a flash of bright lights, Elisse and I awoke, and I was quickly reminded how easy it was to get rest in a hospital – it was 4:00 am and time for the morning vital signs. I remember laying there squinting, half knowing where I was, as the nurse was checking my blood pressure, temperature, and drawing blood from my central line – a catheter surgically inserted to give direct, central access to the heart, where medicine would be delivered and blood withdrawn – this was chemo day 1. Some nurses would try to be as considerate as possible, just turning the light in the bathroom on, providing just enough light to get the job done; however, that was not always the case and more often than not, it was just the opposite.

Trying to wrap my brain around exactly what was happening to me required asking many questions. Some patients don't want any information about what's going on with them while getting treatment, and some want to know everything. I was of the latter and wanted to understand everything and so my education in this new world, that would later become my career and so much more, had now begun. At this stage, it was pretty basic and I was only concerned with my blasts count and absolute neutrophil count (ANC), as blasts indicated remission vs. no response, and ANC (# of neutrophils I had to fight infection) indicated when I could be discharged. Those numbers were the only things I focused on, as I had a new house to enjoy, my wedding to attend, and the rest of my life ahead of me.

At this point, I knew the role of chemotherapy was to rid my body of the cancer cells; however, in doing so, it would also harm and possibly kill cells that were not cancerous. Cancer cells are basically cells that are immortal and divide or multiply at an exponentially faster rate than normal cells that have a preset life cycle. Cancer cells have bypassed this preprogrammed cell death (apoptosis) by utilizing and/or bypassing various pathways, turning on and off certain genes, and using and/or blocking certain proteins. Chemo attacks rapidly dividing cells, which is great for eradicating cancer cells, but not so good for the cells of the gastrointestinal (GI) tract and various other organs which also have rapidly dividing cells. In comes nausea, vomiting, diarrhea, hair loss, organ failure – all side effects of chemo. The ultimate strategy for this treatment was to give chemo for a week to eradicate the cancer, and then stay in the hospital until my body and counts had recovered, which could take several weeks.

During these days in the hospital, I had many visitors, including family, friends, and colleagues. I received countless cards and phone calls from former teachers, family, friends, and friends of friends. It truly is amazing to watch this dynamic unfold before your eyes, as people reach out to make contact, not knowing for sure if this may be the last time they are able to do so. You really start to see what your friends can handle and what they cannot and who can and who cannot. There were friends I had that just couldn't come to grips with what was happening, and I have since lost touch with them over the years, and then there are friends I have grown closer to throughout this ordeal.

The first person we called, after the immediate family was notified, was my college roommate, Bob, who is really more like the brother I never had. At the time Bob was living and working near Midland, Texas which is about a five hour drive to Dallas. Elisse made the call to him as I wasn't able to. Before breaking the news to Bob, Elisse wanted to make sure that he was in a safe position to hear the news. She started out by asking how he was and what he was doing, and he immediately knew something was wrong. Bob is an engineer by trade and someone who thinks in a linear manner, so it didn't take him long to demand to know what was going on and tell her to just spit it out. When she told him the news, he said he was going to get his brother, John, and that they'd see us in five hours. Elisse told him to go to bed and wait until morning to make the trip, but Bob had already made up his mind and there was no stopping him from coming to be there for us that night.

It was good to see him and I was glad he had made the trip, especially since he had with him several items of clothing and some other items he had "borrowed" from me while we were roommates. Amazing thing was that these items had miraculously appeared after I got sick. I thought they had gotten lost during my multiple moves. I still give Bob a hard time about the miraculous resurrection of my belongings to this day.

"Coming clean" seemed to be a recurring theme throughout my stay, as I had another friend, Scott, confess to putting an ice cream sandwich in my fish tank one night after heavily celebrating Texas Tech's defeat over A&M. Scott, like all aggies, is "passionate" about them, and I guess he felt an ice cream sandwich in my fish tank would somehow right some wrong incurred by Tech winning that night. Of course at the time, he profusely denied it. Though here he was in my hospital room now confessing this transgression in front of his mom, his sisters, my nurses, my mom, and Elisse. It was quite amusing to watch to say the least.

My hospital room was also utilized by a friend's ex-girlfriend to stalk him. I don't recall how she knew I was there or how she knew he would be coming to visit, but she camped out in my room for about four hours while she waited for him to show up. Once Mike showed up, she just sat there silently staring at him. Elisse could tell I was exhausted and just wanted to rest, so she broke the awkward silence, and offered to take them to our new house. On the way, not knowing they were broken up, Elisse asked how they were doing, and was awkwardly informed they were no longer a couple. Not much was said during the tour of our new home and Elisse was relieved when they all parted ways that afternoon. Although I was exhausted, these types of visits, or the aftermath of them definitely made my hospital stay less boring and took my mind away from all the uncertainty that lay before me.

As days went by, my mom (my dad was only able to come up on the weekends due to work) and sister, Lori, (had flown in) would stay in my room with me taking notes, asking questions, keeping me company, and playing games, while Elisse would go to work. When Elisse would make her way up to the hospital after work, Lori and my mom would leave and stay at our house. This was the routine until I was discharged. This proved an interesting dynamic for Elisse, my mom, and Lori and would have proven more difficult if not for the European trip we all spent together getting to know each other.

I recall when Lori first showed up. The timing was not the best, as I had just been given a dose of amphotericin, which is an antifungal drug (commonly referred to as "ampho-terrible" by the nurses). My compromised immune system left me vulnerable to a host of microbes and I had developed a fungal infection in my blood, which had spread and been discovered in my eyes upon an eye exam. One of the common effects of amphotericin, aside from killing deadly fungal infections, was tremors. These tremors were so bad they would cause me to bounce on the bed, almost like convulsions and the only remedy was Demerol. I often said Demerol was the absolute best thing about amphotericin, because when the Demerol took effect, I could care less (because I did still care, although a little) about what was going on. So here I was going through one of these tremors, when in walks my sister who hasn't seen me since I was diagnosed, and certainly wasn't expecting to see her little brother in that condition, nor was she expecting her soon to be sister-in-law telling the nurses to get her (my sister) out of the room, but Elisse just didn't want Lori to see me like that without any warning.

Infections were a serious issue with this treatment and any treatment using chemo, because as chemo is eradicating the cancer cells, it is also killing all the good normal cells needed to fight infection – those neutrophils – one of the counts I was concerned with – my ANC. With chemo, the ANC often drops just above zero which translates to hardly any ability to fight infections.

The human body is riddled with bacteria that in a normal person would not pose any risk because it is kept in check by the normal functioning of the immune system; however, with patients undergoing chemo, this normal bacteria can be life-threatening. With little to no immune system, managing infections was achieved via two prongs – growth factor support and intravenous (IV) antimicrobials. GCSF (granulocyte colony stimulating factor), or growth factor support is used to boost the neutrophils that fight infection and is delivered through the IV like all the other medications. Basically it stimulates the marrow to produce those neutrophils that fight infection, but if it's given too soon, it can also stimulate the blasts, so the timing is crucial as to when it's given. Administration of IV antimicrobials (antibacterials, antivirals, antifungals) is the other way infections are managed. Utilizing GCSF coupled with the use of antimicrobials is often the way patients are managed, as was the case in my situation, with the amphotericin I received along with the GCSF. Now the GCSF was great in getting my counts back up, but I sure could tell when it was working, as it caused excruciating, often times debilitating bone pain, originating from the overstimulation of the bone marrow. The bone pain caused from the GCSF injections and the tremors caused from the amphotericin were by far the worst part of my first introduction to cancer treatment.

I was soon beginning to realize just how uncertain all my certainties were becoming, as the second thing I was certain of – being home by Thanksgiving – was missed. This hit me as I was having my first and last Thanksgiving in the hospital, and oh what a Thanksgiving it was. I must say there aren't quite words to accurately express what it's like having Thanksgiving dinner with your family in the hospital with IV medications running through your body while sitting in your hospital bed attached to an IV pole. Although, it definitely wasn't how I was hoping to spend it, that Thanksgiving was probably one of the most thankful Thanksgivings I had up to that point, as here I was in remission from cancer celebrating with my family and well on my way to discharge.

My parents, soon to be in-laws, and Elisse were all there and we had non-hospital homemade turkey, green bean casserole, corn casserole, and potato casserole, all thanks to our moms and Elisse's sister, Laura. Thanksgiving was one of my favorite meals while in the hospital, not that the hospital food was all that bad, just a little monotonous. The other meal that rivaled this one was the Taco Bell dinner my home pastor, John Davenport, drove three hours to deliver to me up from Austin. Now this doesn't mean the Thanksgiving dinner was bad or even comparable to Taco Bell in anyway, it only shows my pure love for Taco Bell at the time. I've matured beyond that now – well a little.

About three quarters of the way through my hospitalization, although unbeknownst to me at the time, a bone marrow transplant physician, Dr. Craig Rosenfeld, came by to talk with me. I had already made up my mind I wasn't doing a transplant, as I had already received the initial report from my post chemo bone marrow biopsy that I was now in remission. In my mind, I was done with this and just waiting for my counts to recover so I could be discharged. Nonetheless, I listened to what he had to say. He informed me that although I was in remission at this point, there was a possibility of relapse and the only known cure was a bone marrow transplant (BMT). He said we would need to wait to see what my chromosomal analysis showed, which would provide a better indication of relapse possibilities in the future. In the meantime, however, he wanted to type Lori and me to see if we were a match. I said sure thing, not a problem, it couldn't hurt, but I knew in my mind I wouldn't need a transplant.

As time went on, the question of should I or shouldn't I have the transplant kept coming up and I must say it was a hard call to make. I was faced with two options at this point. I could (1) receive another round of consolidation chemo after I had recovered from this round, or (2) undergo more intensive chemo and possibly radiation, then transplantation. Being that I was already in remission, and this first round of chemo was pretty much a cake walk, but for the fungal infection and bone pain, consolidation with more chemo didn't sound like too bad an option. On the other hand, what if I were to relapse after the consolidation chemo, would I get a third round, or fourth round, and how many rounds of chemo could my body take before it started shutting down?

Transplantation was an option, but first I would have to find a match. How long would that take? What if my sister didn't match? And the regimens, the regimens used in transplantation could potentially kill me themselves, not to mention the ramifications of rejecting the transplant. My processing and frame of mind at this point was scattered and all over the place. Basically, I could take my chances with chemo alone and just get more rounds of chemo each time if and when I relapsed and potentially live a long somewhat healthy/normal life (except when undergoing chemo), or I could do the transplant for a potential cure and never have to have chemo again, but could quite possibly die while undergoing the transplant. So at age 24, I was having to weigh which option was better – potential lifelong intermittent treatment with death far off, or potential cure with the tradeoff of potential death before I reached 25. This, by far, was going to be the hardest decision I would ever have to make…or so I thought.

Thanksgiving had now come and gone, and although I missed my goal of being home by Thanksgiving, I hadn't missed it by much, as now my doctors were saying my fungal infection had cleared up and with my counts recovering, I would be discharged soon. It even looked as if I was going to be getting out on December 14th – two days before our originally planned wedding date of December 16th. This was exciting news for us, as not only was I going home in about a week, but it looked as if we would be able to get married on the date we had originally planned, although we had about a week to work this out from a logistics standpoint.

Finding a venue to hold the wedding somewhere in the DFW area was the first thing we had to do, as I wasn't cleared to travel too far away from the hospital. Even though my fungal infection had cleared, I still had to get a six hour IV infusion of amphotericin daily for the next three weeks to finish up the six week antifungal course. Additionally, we had to drastically scale back our relatively large wedding to only family and maybe one or two friends each. We, or Elisse rather, started making phone calls to our videographer, photographer, and Pastor Davenport, who mentioned he would give us a pass on the "pre-marital" counseling we were unable to complete due to the rude interruption cancer had made in our plans. He said what we had been through already provided a stronger foundation than anything he would be able to provide. He felt comfortable marrying us without needing any further information to ascertain just how strong our relationship was prior to cancer, and how much stronger this ordeal made it.

Elisse and one of her new friends from work, Lizz, made calls and were able to find a location in downtown Dallas where we could have the wedding and the reception. We picked our witnesses, my dad as best man and Bob for me, and for my wife, her best friend since childhood, Chrystal, whose sister had died from leukemia when they were children, along with another friend, Erin, from back home. Other than our immediate family, those were the only people invited. The wedding went from a $15K occasion with 200+ invited guests to one of about $1200 and about 30 guests. As we were getting closer to discharge and the wedding, we had to get a marriage license, and thankfully Elisse was able to proxy for me at the county clerk's office. One of my nurses took my measurements for the tux, and with that we had managed to "replan" our entire wedding in about a week.

Discharge day was finally upon us now. I had received my six hour antifungal infusion, my vitals were good, my counts were strong and I was ready. The doctors signed me out and a few hours later, my wheelchair and transporter arrived to wheel me outside – a place I hadn't been in 28 days. There, waiting right outside the door of the hospital while waiting for our car to be pulled around, was a gentleman smoking his cigarette – not something I imagined getting a whiff of, fresh off a cancer ward – more irony. Our car was eventually pulled up, I was helped in, and off we went. As we slowly began making our way home, to our new home, I believe that was the first time I broke down realizing what I had just been through and how overjoyed and overwhelmed I was it was all behind me.

When we walked into our new house, which we received keys to on our way to the hospital a month ago, I had immediately realized another benefit of being hospitalized for chemotherapy. Everything was unpacked and our furniture was moved and set up. Elisse, along with family and our friends and their families, had all moved us in while I was in the hospital. Mental note – getting cancer – very effective way to get out of moving.

The first night in our new house was a nice welcomed change, although a bit unnerving at the same time. Although, the nurses coming in the hospital room multiple times throughout the night to check vitals and what not, made it difficult to sleep, it also provided a comfort level I realized I no longer was afforded at home. Nonetheless, sleep came as did the morning along with the home health nurse assigned to administer the six hour IV antifungal infusion. After the infusion was over, the nurse left, and we were off to make the last minute preparations for our wedding the next day. The first stop was to pick up the tuxes, and everything fit well with the exception of the shoes. Although they were size 16 and larger than my normal size 12, they were too tight with all the excess fluid I had from all the IV medications I had been given. My feet were literally coming out of the top of the shoes, but that was the biggest size they had, so we made it work.

The rest of the day for us guys was pretty relaxing, as I was already worn out just from trying on my tux. Needless to say, there wasn't much of a bachelor's party, actually there was no bachelor party. Elisse and her friends spent their day taking care of last minute details and attempting to make flowers for the wedding party.

Thanks to a suggestion my home health nurse made earlier in the morning, we were able to make one more addition to our wedding guest list. It just so happened she had a good friend who played the piano professionally and he was able to play at our wedding with one day's notice. The evening was now upon us and, with Elisse in a hotel room across town and me holding down the fort at our new house, we waited for the morning of December 16, 2000 to come.

A little note–
to say you are in my
thoughts and
prayers today.

I was so shocked and sad when I heard of Ryan's health problems. I too am praying for his complete recovery.

Love. Leona Kodel

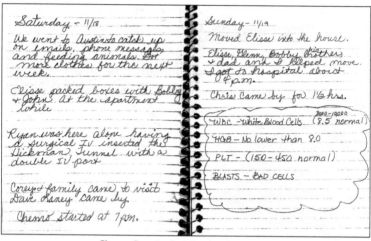

Saturday – 11/18

We went to Austin to catch up on emails, phone messages, and feeding animals. Got more clothes for the next week.

Elisse packed boxes with Bobby + John at the apartment while

Ryan was here alone having a surgical IV inserted the "Hickman" tunnel with a double IV port

Corey + family came to visit. Dave Raney came by.

Chemo started at 1 pm.

Sunday – 11/19

Moved Elisse into the house.

Elisse, Glenn, Bobby, brothers + dad and I helped move. I got to hospital about 4 p.m.

Chris came by for 1½ hrs.

WBC – White Blood Cells (8.5 normal) 5000–10000

HGB – No lower than 8.0

PLT – (150 – 450 normal)

BLASTS – BAD CELLS

Chemo Day 1 – Starting having visitors

Nov. 20, 2000

Dear Elisse;

Your parents told us of Ryan's illness. Very sad but it can be treated and put into remission. We were upset when Anne was diagnosed with Hodgin's Disease. He underwent a lot of treatment and has been in remission

---

God is your strength and shield.
In Him, there is eternal hope.
May He be to you a never-ending source of comfort, hope and peace.

Love
Leona Kobel

I am Amber Schwausch's great-aunt.

Supportive card – people had to tell me who they were in their cards of support, because people I didn't know would still send cards.

I use the term "normal" somewhat loosely, of course.

Hey Ryan,

I'm sorry I couldn't come up with the reels but I've been fighting a cold for 2 weeks, and I don't want to give it to ya! I hope you avoid too bored and giving the Dr.s & nurses too heck of a time. For their sakes, I sent some things to help you pass the time. I wish I was closer so I could come bother you on a regular basis!! Wouldn't that be fun?!

Ryan, I just want you to know that you are in my thoughts and prayers. If you ever need to talk, feel free to give me a call – 24/7!

My mom & dad & brothers also told

More support – friends telling me to call 24/7 no matter what.

Article sent by Elisse's grandmother. Although this article talked about a drug for a different type of leukemia, chronic myeloid leukemia (CML), this drug was the beginning of "targeted therapy" and interestingly enough, the hallmark of a great deal of the study drugs that are currently in clinical trials. As the article states, "...it (drug) is a model for future cancer study because it targets the cause of the disease...". This drug in particular specifically inhibited the tyrosine kinase that produced the BCR/ABL protein which was the driving force for this particular form of leukemia.

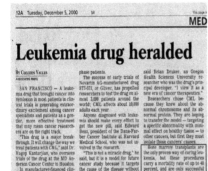

12A Tuesday, December 5, 2000   M

MED

Leukemia drug heralded

BY COLLEEN VALLES
ASSOCIATED PRESS

SAN FRANCISCO — A leukemia drug that brought cancer into remission in most patients in clinical trials is generating extraordinary excitement among cancer specialists and patients as a gentler, more effective treatment that may mean cancer researchers are on the right track.

"This drug is a major breakthrough. It will change the way we treat patients with CML," said Dr. Hagop Kantarjian, who oversees trials of the drug at the MD Anderson Cancer Center in Houston.

In manufacturer-financed clinical trials, more than 90 percent of patients in the first phase of chronic myeloid leukemia saw their cancer go into remission within the first six months of taking the pill, according to result presented Monday at the American Society of Hematology convention.

The drug also appears to be effective in patients in more advanced phases. A study of patients in the second phase of the disease showed more than 90 percent responded positively to treatment, and in 83 percent, the cancer went into remission. The trials involved 530 first-phase and 236 second-

phase patients.

The success of early trials of Novartis AG-manufactured drug STI-571, or Glivec, has propelled researchers to test the drug on almost 3,000 patients around the world; CML affects about 10,000 adults each year.

Anyone diagnosed with leukemia should make every effort to get the new pill, said Edward Benz, president of the Dana-Farber Cancer Institute at Harvard Medical School, who was not involved in the research.

"This is not a miracle drug," he said, but it is a model for future cancer study because it targets the cause of the disease without damaging other cells.

CML, caused by an abnormal protein that is the product of an abnormal chromosome, leads to a huge increase in the number of white blood cells in the body, which can interfere with the functioning of other organs.

Glivec blocks a signal that proteins send out and effectively prevents the abnormal growth and production of other cancerous cells.

"The whole of cancer research has been to identify the differences between cancer cells and normal cells. That's been the goal of cancer research and here it is,"

said Brian Druker, an Oregon Health Sciences University researcher who was the drug's principal developer. "I view it as a new era of cancer therapeutics."

Researchers chose CML because they knew about the abnormal chromosome and its abnormal protein. They are hoping to transfer the model — targeting a specific abnormality with minimal effect on healthy tissue — to other cancers, but first they must isolate those cancers' causes.

Bone marrow transplants are the only proven way of curing leukemia, but these procedures carry a mortality rate of up to 40 percent, and are only successful in 55 percent of cases. Other drugs are used to maintain the health of leukemia patients, but don't decrease the number of white blood cells or help make the blood normal again.

Glivec has been studied on humans for only about two years, so how long it will prolong a patient's life is not yet known. But it has few side effects, and only about 2 percent of patients stop using it because of those side effects.

The drug is expected to hit the market in June. Patients who hope to receive the treatment have to join a clinical trial.

Bone marrow transplants are the
only proven way of curing leukeia,
but these procedures carry a
mortality rate of up to 40 percent,
and are only successful in 55 percent
to 65 percent of cases.

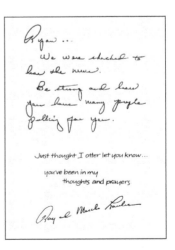

Supportive card from Elisse's grandmother regarding a newspaper article talking about a new drug to treat leukemia. Even though this drug treated (targeted) a different type of leukemia, it demonstrates people still tried to send encouraging news to keep me positive.

11-20-00

I regret to hear of Ryan's health problem. I will keep Ryan in my prayers.
Perhaps we can meet at another time. Sincerely,
Charles Gober

Everybody is thinking about you here, and you are in our prayers.
Sincerely,
Jason and Stacey

Dear Patty and Glen,

Kim has shared with Rich and I the news regarding Ryan's health. Please know that our prayers are with you and your family. I also spoke with your nephew (John). It appears that Ryan is upbeat and is approaching this with a good attitude. I know that we are far away, however if there is anything we can do, please let us know. We think the world of Mark and Kim, Joann and Donna and of course your guys. Most importantly, know that we are there when you need us. May God grant Ryan the strength and words of comfort for you, and especially for Ryan. Our love always,
Rich and Marlene

More supportive cards from friends of extended family
whom I didn't know, yet still reached out offering support

Ryan + family
We will keep you + your family in our prayers. We'll keep close contact with Grandma Mildred. She is a close + dear friend of ours as your Mom + Dad are. Mom will probably have to explain who we are but thats natural. Take care + be good.

Love
Alice

11-24-00

May God give you His peace during this time of illness. Please be assured of our prayers for your full recovery.

Our thoughts and prayers are with you + your family
Love
Allen, Alice + family
Birnbaum

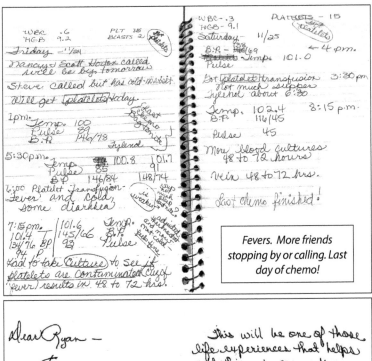

WBC .6
HGB 9.2
PLT 18
BLASTS 2

Friday - 1/24

Nancy & Scott Horton called
will be by tomorrow

Steve called but has cold - won't visit

Will get platelets today.

1pm - Temp. 100
Pulse 89
B.P 146/78
Tylenol

5:30 p.m. Temp. 100.8 101.7
Pulse 85 91
BP 146/84 148/74

6:00 Platelet Transfusion -
Fever and cold,
some diarrhea

7:15 pm. 101.6 Temp.
101.4 T 145/66 BP
134/76 BP 93 Pulse
94 P
Had to take Culture to see if
platelets are Contaminated (cuz of
fever) results in 48 to 72 hrs.

WBC - .3 PLATELETS - 15
HGB - 9.1
Saturday - 11/25
B.P - 138/69 ← 4 pm.
Platelet Temp. 101.0
Pulse

Got platelet transfusion 3:30 pm
Not much supper
Tylenol about 6:30

Temp. 102.4 8:15 p.m.
B.P 116/45

Pulse 45

More blood cultures
48 to 72 hours

Vein 48 to 72 hrs.

Last chemo finished!

> Fevers. More friends
> stopping by or calling. Last
> day of chemo!

Dear Ryan -

*Though you're always
doing nice things for others,
It's time to do
something nice for you,
So relax, take it easy, (as if they
would let you up to do something)
stay comfy and cozy
And before long,
you will feel good as new!*
We are all praying for that!
Hope You're Well Soon

This will be one of those
life experiences that helps
put things in perspective
like love, family & friends &
of course, God. He will see you
through & restore your health.

See what He's done for me.
Happy Thanksgiving!
We'll be thinking of you!
Love,
Bonnie, Dennis,
Jessica, Jeremy
& Joshua

Supportive card from a family in my hometown church I was close with. The
mom had recently come through a battle of breast cancer and offered true words
of support. "...this will be one of those life experiences that helps put things in
perspective..." – how right she was.

Sorry to hear you're
not feeling so great.
Just wanted you
to know that
you're being thought of
and wished
a quick recovery.

Ryan, we are wishing you well.
Your dad was our best man
in our wedding. We also named
our son after your dad.
Miller is a brother to Alec
Birnbaum. We try to keep
up with your family.
Ryan, we are praying for you!
The wedding, the new house.
all things will work out.

Ryan, may all of God's blessing
be with you now and in
the future.

Milton, Guellie, Glen
Albrecht

Supportive card from distant relatives offering support and prayers for the wedding, the new house, and all things working out.

THAT'S A MILLION BUCKS AFTER TAXES!

get well soon + remember if you
win the lottery don't take the big
sum, take it in pieces, Cody.

get well and feel better soon, be happy.
say hi to everybody. Grow back your hair.
Kelsey Rene Woelfel. love u.

I love you, you know your my
favorite cousin, ♡ Kaci

Support from cousins

WITH ALL OUR LOVE,

LIBERTY HILL INTERMEDIATE SCHOOL

Support from Mom's work and middle school I attended growing up

Hope you know
that many thoughts
and prayers are with you

We just want you to know
our prayers are with you and
if you need anything at all
we are only a phone call
away! Take care +
God Bless!
Love,
Monica +
Cory
Wegele

Now's the time to get well!

Ryan –
We were so sorry to hear
about your illness. You have
been in our prayers daily. As
a cancer survivor myself, I can
understand and relate to the
exhausting and traumatic difficulties
you have experienced over the past
few weeks. Just remember, you are
in the Lord's hands.

Support from other cancer survivors

WBC. - 10.4   PLT- 149
HGB - 9.3

~~Tuesday~~ 9/12/12

Pastor Davenport came up.

BP. 117/48
Pulse 76
Temp. 97.7

Dr. Joseph opthalmologist said Ryan has a scar on his right retina and some blood in his right eye - maybe broken blood vessels

BP. 110/52
Pulse 80
Temp. 98.3

Note regarding a scar tissue on my retina most likely
occurring from one of those "non-studying" nights in college.
Drinking was involved as well as Bob sucker-punching me.

Ryan,
  You continue to be in our prayers on Sundays during our worship services & again during our staff meetings. We pray that God will touch your life with a sense of peace & healing.
  Your Friends in Christ,
  Abiding Presence Lutheran Church

Stained glass window, 12 feet high,
Abiding Presence Lutheran Church, San Antonio, Texas

Supportive card from church
in San Antonio

Get Well Soon!

Ryan, your name is in prayers all over San Antonio. And we wanted you to know that everyone cares about you. Get stronger so we can come up there.
  Love, Granny & Paw Paw

More prayers and support
from San Antonio

...till you can come out and play.

We've completely depleted HEB's supply of "Get Well" cards - guess I need to shop elsewhere (don't tell hubby). Hope this week is better than last week for you. You remain in our prayers, cutie.
Elisse tells me you can now shave with your hand - that would have some advantages I think. The girls were in our church christmas pagent yesterday, and Saturday we had Margi's birthday party here - just girls! I'm still finding sticky stuff in odd places. Margi's Barbie collection has grown once again!
  God bless you,
    Love,
    Mark, Kim, Margi, & Elissa

Ryan-

I saw this card & thought of you. The strength you possess will carry you through all of life's tough moments. Remember that, and always keep your positive outlook.

    Love,
    Laura

Supportive card from Elisse's sister

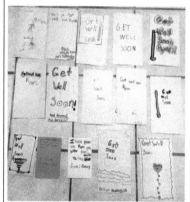

Dear Ryan...

Hope you are doing well. Give our love to your Mom and Dad as well as Elisse!

We pray for you each day.

    Roy & Marsha Fowler

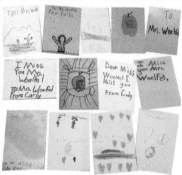

*Cards from my Mom's
3rd grade class*

Dear Patty
We are praying for Ryan and your whole family during this crisis. Please let us know if there is anything we can do. Hang in there, girl.

I just want you to know that I'm thinking about you.

Love,
Mike, Chris & Katie

Wishing you
a holiday season
filled with
beautiful moments.

Dear Erin —   12/2
Thank you so much for attending my bridal shower! I really like all of the baking items and can't wait until Ryan is home so I can cook for him! Thanks again you're GREAT!

as always,
Ryan & Susse

Dear Ryan,
I'm sure this time of your life reminds you of a book *Does Third Grade Last Forever?* (does this trial last forever)? We are praying that it is over soon and never comes again. It will be so good to have you back in circulation again. We are also praying for Elise, who is by your side, and your sister, Lori, and your parents.

Hey, Ryan.
I thought of you when I saw this one so I couldn't resist but send it. I really appreciate

Get well soon!

your family keeping me informed via e-mail. Know that you and your family are in my prayers. I know God is taking care of you, and though I don't understand everything, I know He has a perfect plan.
Please keep smiling your friendly smile and know all of the embarrassing moments are building character (like you don't have enough already)!

Blessings,
Jessica Halvorson

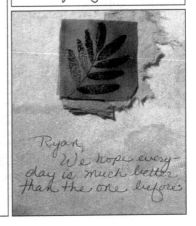

Ryan,
We hope everyday is much better than the one before.

Consultation Note
New Patient

Craig S. Rosenfeld, MD
Texas Cancer Center
at Medical City Dallas
7777 Forest Lane, D-220
Dallas, TX 75230

Patient:	Woefel, Ryan	MedRecNum:	NP
Dictate:	12-6-00	Visitation:	12-5-00
Tscribe:	12-6-00 lje		

I was kindly asked by Dr. Stone to evaluate this 24-year-old with recently-diagnosed AML for transplant options. His history of present illness is outlined below:

DATE: **EVENT:**

10/99   Onset of bleeding gum, ecchymosis and sore throat.

11/14/00   The patient was in Columbus, Ohio on business. A CBC reveals a white count of 42,000 with 62% blasts. The Hgb = 8.9 and platelet count = 11,000. He was given a platelet transfusion.

11/15/00   The patient was referred to Dr. Stone and admitted to Medical Center of Plano. Physical examination was remarkable for numerous ecchymoses. Neither gingival hyperplasia or splenomegaly is noted. CBC reveals a white count of 57,200 with 42% blasts. The Hgb = 8.4 and platelets = 50,000. Chemistry was significant for an LDH = 826. A marrow performed on 11/16/00 was 100% cellular and was replaced by blasts. Auer rods were not identified. Flow cytometry suggests a monocytic leukemia. Myeloperoxidase was positive. Cytogenetics reveal 46,XY,del(7q),del(16q), t(16;18)(p11.2;p11.32)[14]46,XY[1].

11/16/00   The patient was started on 7+3 (Idarubicin).

12/4/00   A repeat marrow is 5% cellular without obvious leukemic replacement. Positive blood cultures for yeast.

PAST MEDICAL HISTORY:

MEDICATIONS: (Preadmission) None.

ALLERGIES: None.

FAMILY HISTORY: Negative for leukemia, lymphoma or aplastic anemia.

Page 2

SOCIAL HISTORY: The patient is engaged. He recently started work for iNET Technologies. He does not drink or smoke.

SIBLINGS: One sister (Laurie).

PHYSICAL EXAMINATION: Deferred.

IMPRESSION:
High-risk FAB-M for AML, undergoing initial induction chemotherapy.

RECOMMENDATIONS:

This 24-year-old has high-risk AML. He is identified as having high-risk disease by having both a 7q- and complex cytogenetic abnormalities. For this reason, he should be considered as a transplant candidate early in the course of his disease.

In a 90-minute meeting, I reviewed the history of present illness, options for therapy and specific procedures, expectations and potential complications of allogeneic transplantation for AML. I told Mr. Woefel that a chance of chemotherapy curing his disease was < 10%.

I reviewed the procedures to identify an HLA-identical sibling. Mr. Woefel has one sibling (a sister). I then explained that alternative donors could be obtained from either the National Marrow Donor Program or Cord Blood Registry.

I then discussed the following procedures: high-dose chemotherapy or chemo/radiotherapy, infusion of stem cells and possible need for transfusions and antibiotics and hospitalization.

Concerning potential complications, I told Mr. Woefel the major complication of allogeneic transplantation was acute graft-versus-host disease. I told him that the risk of acute graft-versus-host disease depended on the HLA match of the donor.

Concerning timing, I suggested that Mr. Woefel be transplanted early in his course.

Craig S. Rosenfeld, M.D.

cc: Scott Stone, MD
3705 W. 15th Street
Plano, Texas 75075

Consultation note from bone marrow transplant doctor – Craig Rosenfeld.

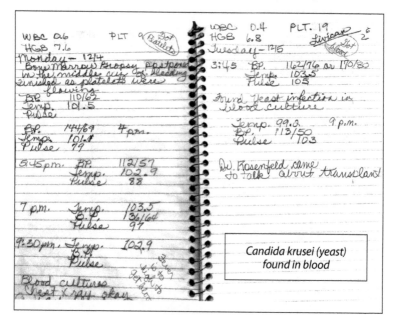

Candida krusei (yeast) found in blood

December 11, 2001

Dear Elisse & Ryan,

The days leading up to your wedding were long and arduous, but it's amazing how fast this past year has gone by. If wishing could make it so, your beginning would have been much smoother and less complicated. But the trials you endured this past year will not only strengthen your marriage, but also help to prepare you for whatever lies ahead. Life is always full of surprises.

Dad and I are enjoying our vacation, taking one day at a time and just doing whatever we feel like doing that day. I got most of my Christmas cards and letters finished yesterday, but ran out of cards. I ordered more cards a couple weeks ago, but as they haven't arrived yet, I may have to get another box at the store this week so I can finish them up and get them mailed in time to arrive before Christmas. Dad has gone to the barber to get his hair cut this morning, as I sit here trying to finish up the last of the Christmas card list. Chaplin has been ignoring us the past couple of days and acts like it's no big deal that we haven't gone to work this week. I don't know yet when we are coming to Plano, but hopefully, dad will decide soon so we can make plans. My eye surgery is scheduled for December 19th.

Well, better close and get this to the mailbox.

Love, Mom

Words of encouragement from Elisse's mother

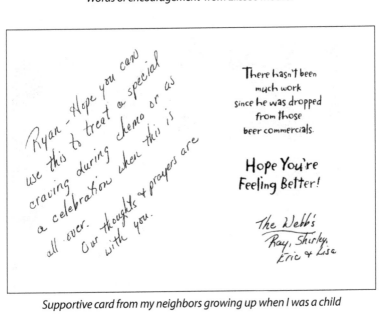

Ryan - Hope you can use this to treat a special craving during chemo or as a celebration when this is all over. Our thoughts & prayers are with you.

There hasn't been much work since he was dropped from those beer commercials.

Hope You're Feeling Better!

The Webb's
Ray, Shirley,
Eric & Lisa

Supportive card from my neighbors growing up when I was a child

```
MEDICAL CENTER OF PLANO     BILLING DATE     PAGE  34
3901 W 15TH                    12/28/00
PLANO, TX  75075-7738
(972) 596-6800                ADMITTED      DISCHARGED
                              11/15/00       12/14/00
```

NDC/CPT-4/ HCPCS	QTY	SERVICE DESCRIPTION	CHARGES
A6258	1	TEGADERM 4" X 4"	12.25
A6258	1	TEGADERM 4" X 4"	12.25
A6258	1	TEGADERM 4" X 4"	12.25
A6258	1	TEGADERM 4" X 4"	12.25
A6258	1	TEGADERM 4" X 4"	12.25
		SUBTOTAL:	128.00
J9211	6	IDAMYCIN 5 MG	5560.08
J9100	3	CYTOSAR 100MG/0.2 VIAL	90.85
J9211	6	IDAMYCIN 5 MG	5560.08
J9100	3	CYTOSAR 100MG/0.2 VIAL	90.85
J9211	6	IDAMYCIN 5 MG	5560.08
J9100	3	CYTOSAR 100MG/0.2 VIAL	90.85
J9100	3	CYTOSAR 100MG/0.2 VIAL	90.85
J9100	3	CYTOSAR 100MG/0.2 VIAL	90.85
J9100	3	CYTOSAR 100MG/0.2 VIAL	90.85
J9100	3	CYTOSAR 100MG/0.2 VIAL	90.85
		SUBTOTAL:	17316.19
99221	1	INTL NUTR SERV LOW COM	39.00
99232	1	SBSQ NUTRCARE MOD COMP	32.50
99232	1	SBSQ NUTRCARE MOD COMP	32.50
99232	1	SBSQ NUTRCARE MOD COMP	32.50
		SUBTOTAL:	136.50

```
          TOTAL ANCILLARY CHARGES        103505.70

                  TOTAL CHARGES          119455.70
                       PAYMENTS                .00
                    ADJUSTMENTS                .00
                        BALANCE          119455.70
```

*$119,455.70 – Hospital bill for one months stay,
chemo, drugs, care, and remission!*

CHAPTER 4: THE WEDDING

With the ring of the doorbell at 6 a.m. came the morning of the wedding along with the home health infusion nurse to begin my six hour IV antifungal infusion, and my new best friend – Demerol. Once the infusion ended, I was disconnected from the IV pump and we began our day. It was a little after noon and the wedding was set to begin around 6 p.m. that evening. Pastor Davenport soon arrived, and asked if I wanted anymore Taco Bell. After cracking a few jokes about that, we all headed to the study to catch some of the football game that was on. Coincidentally, Elisse's maid of honor, Crystal, had a brother-in-law who happened to be playing in the game and had just made a big play. We watched some more of the game, and before we knew it, it was about time to head to the wedding venue.

I recall everyone asking if I was getting nervous or getting cold feet, and I remember thinking I hadn't really had much time to think about getting cold feet, or if I was nervous, as I was just hoping and praying that Elisse wouldn't end up a widow before she reached her mid-twenties. Although I was in remission, I still had a big decision ahead of me that would affect all of us in the near future – to transplant or not to transplant, and that question consumed most of my thoughts at that time.

Bob drove me to the wedding and as we were pulling into the parking lot at the place we were getting married, the Pegasus Room, a guy coming out of the parking lot took up most of the entry way. Bob started yelling, "Man – come-on now – who's this jackass – look at this guy!" I looked up to see "this guy" waiving at us and when I realized who it was, I started laughing.

After catching my breath, I said, "That's Elisse's dad!" Bob and I still joke about that today, but no matter what Bob says about his parking lot maneuvering, he's great. I don't know how many father-in-laws would rub lotion on their son-in-law's dry, cracked, and scaly feet, which he did while visiting during my next hospitalization.

Once we parked, we got out of the car and went inside and I introduced Bob to my soon to be father-in-law and once again we started laughing. We made it down to the bar area to have a few drinks and visit with some of the guests, until it was time to get ready for the wedding.

Our wedding venue was split in three levels with a bar downstairs. The main level consisted of the room we were getting married in and a reception area in the back. The changing area was upstairs on the third level, and this is where Elisse descended down a flight of stairs rivaling those in the Titanic movie. Just like with watching the movie, it was hard holding back the tears, although this moment was far more emotional.

With the way the room was set up, the small wedding party, Elisse, her two friends (Chrystal and Erin), my dad, Bob, and Pastor Davenport were situated in the middle of the room with our family surrounding us. As Pastor Davenport began quoting scripture and providing some of the back story regarding Elisse and I, he mentioned how I had been healed by the "Great Physician," and how through "Divine Design" this day, although threatened by cancer, had still been allowed to happen. I remember although we were surrounded by family and very few friends, it seemed like only Elisse and I were really there. Everything else was just kind of off in the background and I could barely even focus on what the pastor was saying, except when he mentioned the words, "till death do you part" – those words never had any real meaning to me prior to that day at that moment, and I could tell from Elisse's tear-filled eyes, she was thinking the same thing I was. It was an emotional service and I don't believe there was a dry eye in the place, including the people working the event.

At the conclusion of the wedding, we preceded to the back area of the room to have the reception. The place provided the guest with two choices for the main course, either chicken or steak, with salad and champagne. They also provided two cakes, one white wedding cake and a groom's Texas Tech Double T cake.

The speeches were all memorable but I think the one my father gave was the best. He said he hoped Elisse and I had a much better marriage and life than he and my mother had, which didn't quite come out the way he meant it to. He quickly qualified his statement, saying he and my mother had a wonderful marriage and life together, he was just hoping ours would even surpass theirs. The owners of the "Pegasus Room" said we were their first ever wedding and we all felt it went great. Now of course it was time for the honeymoon, which would actually have to wait, as I was still having to get the six hour IV antifungal infusion the next morning, but we still had the wedding night ahead of us.

Our wedding night was unlike that of any I could have ever imagined and not because of the great wild heated sex – it was actually not only because of the lack of sex, but also because I wasn't expecting to play matchmaker on our wedding night. You absolutely cannot have a wedding without someone in the wedding party hooking up, or at the very least, one member trying to hook up with another, and this was the case with ours. As we were on our way out of the reception, Bob was asking me to try to hook him up with Elisse's friend who had come down for the wedding, not the married one – the other one, Erin. I lived with Bob for many years, and he was like a brother to me, so I knew this would be a tall order, but I told him I would try my best. We decided to catch a late movie and see what would happen. I intervened as best I could, but as things usually go in these wedding party hookup scenarios, and much like they did for Elisse and I that evening, Bob saw no action that night except for what happened on the movie screen.

After the movie, Elisse and I checked in to one of the high-rise hotels (a wedding present from Lori) in downtown Dallas for our wedding night, and as I said it was quite memorable. It was pretty late when we checked in, because the movie was a long one. We were both exhausted. Even throughout the wedding, I was a bit unstable on my feet, and they were killing me, as they were bulging out of the size 16 shoes I was in. As I removed the rest of my clothing, I was swollen all over and looked like one big trunk not able to really distinguish my ankle from my thigh, as I was one size all the way down – BIG. Being on my feet all day after getting the six hour infusion led to pretty significant edema (swelling), from all the excess fluid I was taking in. I think we finally passed out from pure exhaustion, and not the good kind.

The next few days were all about recovery, relaxing, and trying to get my strength back. I finally finished with my antifungal infusion on Christmas Eve (early Christmas present) and now I felt free. No more having to get hooked up to an IV pole and no more bags of meds. What an exhilarating feeling and a true realization of some of the simple things we take for granted. Although everything was behind me at this point, for the most part, I was still faced with the decision to transplant or not to transplant, and I had pretty much made up my mind.

I was strong and getting stronger now. I had made it through this round of chemo without any real complications. Induction was a cake walk so to speak, especially given how bad I had heard chemo was. I never really experienced any nausea or other GI toxicities, and with the exception of the bone pain from the Neupogen and side effects from treating the fungal infection, it was really a non-event. I figured I would rather take my chances with further rounds of chemo, should I relapse and live a long life that way. This option seemed much more attractive than taking a chance on transplantation and facing a strong possibility of immediate death from the preparatory regimen in the immediate future. I was pretty much set with my decision, especially given the fact that all I had heard about transplantation was how horrible it was and there wasn't even a guarantee it would work. Then with the "bring bring" of the phone, everything I knew for sure and was certain about, was again about to change.

On the other end of the phone was Dr. Rosenfeld's transplant coordinator. She explained to me my cytogenetics (chromosomal analysis) had come back and what it showed was that I had very complex chromosomal abnormalities and when I asked what exactly that meant, Dr. Rosenfeld got on the phone. He explained that with chemotherapy alone and no transplantation, I had a 95% chance of relapse. I explained I was in remission now though and felt great and asked about waiting to see if I relapse and then do the transplant. He explained doing the transplant while in first remission offered the best chance of survival and waiting until relapse would increase my mortality and morbidity by almost 20%, reducing my chance for survival from 65% to approximately 45%. Although this was horrible news for me, as I wanted nothing to do with a transplant, it was good because it made my decision easy. I was now 100% on board with transplantation. The other thing I found out in this phone call, which was icing on the cake, was my sister and I matched perfectly – a 6 for 6 match.

Bone marrow transplantation is quite different from solid organ transplantation, (e.g., heart, lung, kidney, liver, etc.), in many ways. One in particular is the matching. With solid organ transplantation, one has to be concerned with the recipient's body rejecting the organ. However, in bone marrow transplantation, one is concerned with the graft (donor bone marrow) rejecting the body, as it is the donor's bone marrow that houses the new immune system that will be transplanted. It's quite a different story when the very thing that's being transplanted can consider the body it's being transplanted into as foreign and starts attacking it.

The matching is based on the body's Human Leukocyte Antigen (HLA) system. By today's standards, matching is done predominantly on a 12-match system, and at the time Lori and I were being matched, a perfect match was based on a 6-match system. The HLA system is a very complex one which I believe we now know, or rather have identified > 400 HLA factors. However, it's not known to what significance all of these antigens play in the role of matching. So, then why is 6 the magic number? At this point, it was known these 6 factors play a significant role in how well donors and recipients match. The antigens are called HLA A, B, and Dr, with one group coming from an individual's mother and the other group coming from the father. This system has been genetically passed down through the ages as it is part of our biology, so the combinations are numerous. However, with siblings sharing the same parents, there is a 25% chance of getting the same HLA match, regardless of the number of siblings. So when I heard my sister and I were a perfect 6 for 6 match, I realized how blessed we were, and the words "divine design" like I heard in our wedding, came rushing back.

Even though I was terrified of transplant, at least I didn't have to make the difficult decision of to transplant or not to transplant, as my cytogenetics did that for me. Now I needed to look ahead and process this new challenge. In the next few weeks, I began making preparations. During my induction chemo, my mom pretty much moved in with us, or rather Elisse, as I was in the hospital the whole time, and don't get me wrong, she was a big help. Now however, Elisse and I were beginning this new phase in our lives, and though we appreciated all my mom had done, we wanted to be on our own as much as possible.

I knew my mom would want to be up here for the duration of my transplant. My parents came up one weekend and while Elisse was away from the house, I had "the talk" with them. It was a very emotional and unpleasant conversation. We were sitting in the back room looking at the pool when I braved the conversation. I explained how appreciative we were for my parents and mom coming up and helping while I was undergoing chemo, but as newlyweds Elisse and I wanted to spend as much time together as possible. Although my mom being up here would be a big help, we didn't want her to move in for the entire duration. I further explained – this was the hardest thing for me to get out – if the worst thing happened to me and I didn't make it and died, I wanted to spend as much "alone" time with Elisse as possible. My parents and I had enjoyed 24 years together, but Elisse and I had only the past two years. I felt it wasn't fair for Elisse to split the precious time she had with me with my parents, in case these were my last days here. It was very hard explaining this to my parents and having them see it from our point of view – we had to face the possibility that Elisse could be a widow in less than a month and we wanted time to spend together alone. As someone who wasn't a parent at the time, I didn't realize just how crazy, preposterous, and difficult that request was for my parents to get from their son.

Of course, we didn't expect, or want them to stay away until I was all clear and out of the hospital, we just didn't want them staying with us the whole time. Although it took some time to find some middle ground, we were able to make a compromise. In the beginning, at the very least, they would come up on the weekends only, unless there were complications, or something came up where we needed them…little did we know how soon this would be the case.

Transplant time was rapidly approaching and we were at Dr. Rosenfeld's office having our consult visit. This was a family event, as he had only talked briefly with me in the hospital room when I was undergoing chemo. Now that we were moving forward down this path, he was going into detail, covering all that would be taking place. We discussed expectations, including what my chances of survival were, so it was important for my family to be there. He began to explain about stem cells and pluripontent stem cells and hematopoetic stem cells and cancer and the science behind how all this comes together to provide a cure to the leukemia that was wreaking havoc in my body. What I was in store for, no matter how well he prepared us, didn't come close to what I experienced. I had no idea I was beginning the hardest, yet strangest and also the most crucial journey of my life.

Let's start with pluripotent and hematopoetic stem cells, like Dr. Rosenfeld did. Everybody has cells in their body and we all know that, but all cells are derived from other cells, and those cells from other cells, and this cycle repeats until death. Pluripotent stem cells are the beginning cells, cells that have not differentiated into their genetically defined functioning cells. Each system has its own beginning cells, or stem cells. Embryonic stem cells, which are often in the news and immersed in controversy, are the very early cells that differentiate, or can be programmed or engineered to differentiate into any cell they are genetically predisposed to do, or synthetically altered to do (e.g., cardiac, epithelial, muscular etc.). Mesenchymal stem cells are the stem cells that give rise to cells that form the skin and linings of the mucus membranes of the organs and GI tract. Hematopoietic stem cells are those stem cells that give rise to the cells developed in the bone marrow, which produce red blood cells, platelets, and white blood cells. These cells, derived from hematopoietic stem cells, that develop into the red blood cells, platelets, and white blood cells, were where the root of my malignancy lay. The purpose of chemo is to kill the cancer and in my case, the cancer was in my bone marrow.

Though the chemo did its job and put me in remission, my cytogenetics revealed I would relapse, and that's because I had altered DNA, or genetic code. This altered DNA would give rise to malignant clones in my bone marrow, which would rapidly reproduce more malignant clones leading to eventual relapse. The only way to rid my body of these malignant clones was to kill them with stronger chemo and radiation. This stronger treatment would effectively, not only suppress my bone marrow and therefore immune system, but it would kill it to the point where it would not recover on its own and I would essentially die, without the aid of stem cell rescue – in walks my sister.

Lori was living in England at the time of my diagnosis. "Mad Cow" disease was a big problem in England so blood products from there were generally not allowed in the US. Certain exceptions were allowed and Dr. Rosenfeld said my situation would qualify, but they still needed to work through the red tape. My sister's bone marrow was a perfect match to mine, so risk of rejection was slim to none; however, the risk was still there as my sister and I are clearly not identical.

In order to transfer Lori's bone marrow to me, she would undergo a marrow harvesting procedure. This procedure is a day surgery requiring general anesthesia, so that the bone marrow can be extracted from the lower back (hip region). Lori's procedure would be done by multiple doctors inserting needles into her back to penetrate the bone reaching the marrow and then simultaneously these doctors would aspirate her marrow out of her and inject it into a bag.

After the bag was filled with enough of Lori's life-saving bone marrow, it would then be processed and taken to my room and hung from an IV pole to drip similar to a blood transfusion. Once inside my blood stream, Lori's bone marrow, through biological design, would find its way to my bones where it would take root and start functioning as if it were my own. All the cells needed to live (i.e., red blood cells, white blood cells, and platelets), along with the immune system would be recreated. This process – engrafting – wouldn't occur over night. Engrafting can take weeks and it is the most critical time with the highest risk of death from infection because during the engrafting phase of transplant, a patient has no immune system (i.e., no white blood cells or neutrophils). Other risks include bleeding out internally or externally – due to no platelets, and hypoxia (not enough oxygen in blood) due to no red blood cells or hemoglobin. These were just the potential risks of death from having low blood counts due to the intensive chemo and radiation. There was also risk of death from my body going into multi-organ failure and not being able to process the intensive regimen of therapy I was about to undergo.

Radiation was the other part of my intensive treatment regimen, and because leukemia is in the bone marrow and bone marrow is in bones and bones are all throughout the body, my whole body would be going through radiation – total body irradiation (TBI), not just one local site, as is often the case with solid tumor malignancy such as breast, lung, brain, etc.

Around the time of World War II, tests were done to determine the amount of radiation someone could tolerate before death. These tests gave rise to studying bone marrow transplantation as a way to provide treatment and a rescue from the aftermath of nuclear war. Through these tests, it was learned an adult male can handle about 500cGy of radiation before going into bone marrow failure. This was an important number, because as part of my treatment plan, I would be receiving 1350cGy of total body irradiation. This amount of radiation would, without a doubt, not only kill my cancer and any lingering cancer cells missed by the chemo, but also kill me had I not had the ability to be rescued with replacement marrow from my sister. These strong, super-intense toxic treatments cause bone marrow failure, which normally would lead to death; however, bone marrow failure is not a problem. On the contrary, it's the goal in this situation. With leukemia, the bone marrow is malignant and thus failing already, with the exception of the malignant clone that keeps thriving and dividing, wreaking havoc.

Initially, we were concerned about the intensity of the regimen, but Dr. Rosenfeld assured us it was appropriate due to the aggressive nature of my disease and tolerable because I was a healthy 24 year-old. Though Dr. Rosenfeld felt this was the right regimen for me, he informed us it would most likely kill someone in their 50's. We then moved on to the next part of the conversation – transplant aftermath.

There are three main types of bone marrow or stem cell transplants:

1. Allogeneic – from another person;
2. Autologous – from one's self;
3. Synergenic – from one's twin.

Often times an allogeneic transplant is the optimal choice, but unfortunately, it is not always an option. One of the main risks with allogeneic transplantation is Graft Versus Host Disease (GVHD), where the "graft," is the transplanted stem cells from the donor, and the "host" is the recipient. This occurs because the immune system is built in the bone marrow and since it is the bone marrow being transplanted, it recognizes the host as foreign. The newly transplanted immune system then starts performing its biological function of attacking and ridding the body of foreign objects. This is the reason why matching is so critical and even with a perfect match, GVHD can still occur, as there are many more HLA factors at play than the mere six that are matched when undergoing allogenic transplantation. Since it's the donor stem cells (the graft) that sees the recipient (the host) as foreign, GVHD can attack and affect any organ (e.g., the skin, eyes, GI tract, lungs, liver, etc.).

There are two types of GVHD, acute and chronic. Acute GVHD (aGVHD) can generally occur anytime in the first 100 days post-transplant, whereas Chronic GVHD (cGVHD) can occur at any time after day 100 post-transplant. These pre-defined definitions of acute vs. chronic GVHD dependent on number of days post-transplant, are of course generalities, as cGVHD can also occur in the first 100 days, and aGVHD can also occur after day 100. There can be an overlap and definitions are now looking more at the organ system involved with GVHD to classify it either as acute vs. chronic, rather than merely looking at day 100 as being the defining factor.

Another possibility with allogeneic transplants is graft rejection, which basically occurs when the host rejects the graft. This can often occur if the regimen wasn't strong enough to kill the host's bone marrow (immune system). Essentially the patient's own immune system destroys the transplanted cells and this is usually the cause, if the patient hasn't engrafted by d25 or so, post-transplant.

Aside from rejection, either from the graft rejecting the body, or vice versa, the other main risks associated with transplantation are secondary malignancies (cancers), and long-term latent organ damage. Secondary malignancies can potentially occur because the very treatment (chemo/radiation) used to kill the leukemia and bone marrow are mutagenic intercalaters, meaning it intercalates, or breaks DNA up and mutates, or changes it, which is the root cause of cancer, generally speaking. Long-term latent organ damage occurs from the mere treatment regimens used to kill the cancer, as they are very toxic to the cancer as well as the organs. This toxicity can result in premature aging, hypertension, hyperlipidemia, cardiovascular disease, osteoporosis, pulmonary fibrosis, and many other diseases.

After, explaining all of the side effects and potential hurdles I could be facing in the future, that is if I made it through the treatment and had a future, the last bit of information Dr. Rosenfeld gave us was my chances of survival. Taking into account my youth, the aggressive nature of my leukemia, the match grade of my sister and me, my current health in spite of the leukemia – my number – 65%. A little more than 50% chance of surviving was a lot better than the 5% chance I had without the transplant, so I was sold and signed the consents to get the process started.

It was about a week after Christmas and I was scheduled to be admitted to begin chemo and radiation in about a month; however, first I would need to get another bone marrow biopsy to ensure I was still in remission. If I was not in remission, then all bets were off and transplant would be postponed, or perhaps even canceled. My bone marrow biopsy did in fact reveal I had remained leukemia free – things were looking well. I was anxious but ready.

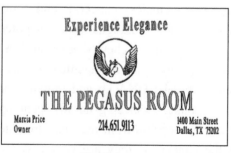

Wedding venue

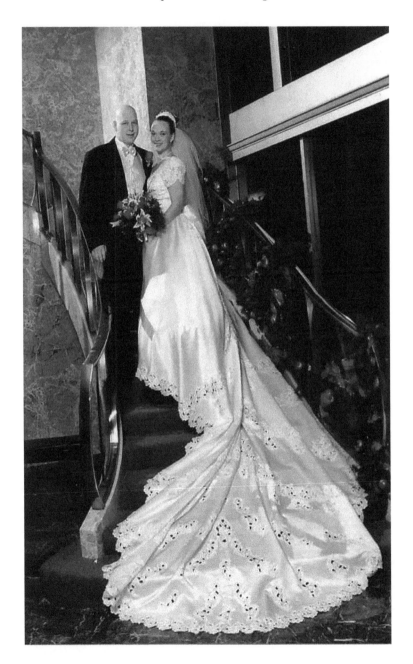

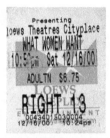

Presenting
loews Theatres Cityplace
WHAT WOMEN WANT
10:59pm Sat 12/16/00
ADULT $6.75

RIGHT 13

12/16/00   10:24pm

*Wedding night movie; Bob's
chance to make a move on
Elisse's bridesmaid*

Ryan & Elisse —
Just a short note to thank you for
the generous check you gave after your
wedding. I was/am honored to be one of
your pastors and so enjoyed the celebration
@ the Pegasus Room. Thanks again.
I know the bone marrow adventure
is on the horizon — we keep Lori in our
prayers, too. Hold on tight to one another
and I'll look forward to seeing you soon.
Peace
Pastor John Davenport

*Words of encouragement from
our Pastor after the wedding*

This is a card I found in a
stack of cards our ladies group
is collecting for St. Jude's
Ranch for children.
It is such a lovely verse
I wanted to share it with
you. I hope you enjoy it as
much as I did.
Love Ya'
Grandma

Ryan & Elisse

May Christ,
whose birth we celebrate,
bless you and those you love
with peace and happiness.

We celebrate your marriage
What a surprise when pastor announced it
in church! We pray for your continued
healing, Ryan, and a wonderful marriage
the album

for those of you who don't know me, this is ryan, lon's brother. i just wanted to say thanks so much for all of your prayers, cards, and words of encouragement. without those things, especially the prayers, i strongly believe i would still be in hospital today. anyway, everything is going great. as most of you now know i have now married my best friend by far, elisse from conroe tx, and life is going good. it is the best feeling in the world to be out of the hospital and have my life somewhat back to normal. this disease that i have, that is now gone, is nothing more than a curve ball that life has thrown me. it really helps to know the support system that one has when times become rough. some of you i have never known, but yet you have taken me into your family prayers, and i thank you for that. if anything, this disease has put things into perspective. it shows how precious life is, and how ridiculous it is to get tied up in everyday problems that arise. even though i got this disease, i still know there are others out there who are far worse than me, who i pray for. the most current update is that i today finished my last bit of antibiotics, and have no need for a home nurse. i have an appointment with my doctor on the dec. 28th to discuss further treatment, which is currently looking like one more and final round of chemo sometime in january. right now i am in remission, and the doctors all said that i came through this first round a perfect as anyone could have asked for. i sincerely believe that is because of all the prayers that yall and others have sent out. some of you have asked where elisse and me are registered; we are registered at target and dillards. sorry to those who feel left out of the wedding, but we are going to have a renewal of vows sometime in the near future that will go on just how we originally planned the first one. i can't say enough how thankful i am for all of you, and may God be with each and every one of you and your family. thanks again, and have a good christmas, because this is by far the best one Ive ever had. thanks again.

ryan

ps: sorry about the lowercase typing, but it's late, and it's much easier for me to type without having to use the shift key. thanks again. if anyone has any questions feel free to ask, and please pass this note along to anyone that i might have missed. thanks again.

*My "thank-you email" to all those who sent support
and who I was able to reach via email*

Blood Drive Successful

"It makes me feel good when I think I can help," Carolyn Schubert said upon setting up an appointment for giving blood. "I donate frequently, so I just decided I'd come up and do so again," said Gary Kurio following his donation. "I can't donate blood since I visited in a Mexico state where malaria was present; however, I will volunteer my time to assist with registration," said Flo Ritter. These were some of the comments heard and the feeling of camaraderie and Christian support expressed. Some forty to fifty people (members as well as non-members) showed up on January 6 to assist and donate blood as a benefit for Zion member Ryan Woelfel. Ryan was recently diagnosed with leukemia and is currently being prepared for a bone marrow transplant. His sister will donate her bone marrow for this procedure. What a heart-wrenching story! Keep them in your prayers.

Teenagers, middle-aged couples and some elderly (whose names will remain anonymous) walked up the steps into the mobile van, climbed on a reclining table, stretched out an arm and within a short period of time had made their contribution. The grateful Woelfel family was present and Mom, too, contributed her blood. Upon expressing thanks, Ryan's father stated "It takes ten pints of blood to make one unit of platelets" and Ryan has needed several units of platelets, as well as whole blood. It is anticipated he will need many more. Perhaps in the not too distant future another drive can be scheduled. This will provide others the opportunity to donate who were unable to do so the first time around.

Donors wanting to know their blood type may call the Scott & White Blood Center at 254/724-2430 or toll free 1/877/724-9181.

The members of the Zion Health Cabinet wish to thank everyone who participated in making our first blood drive such a success. A total of thirty-four pints of blood were accepted for use. A big thank you is also extended to those individuals who registered but for some valid reason were unable to donate. Thanks to the AAL group for furnishing refreshments.

Mimi Kalmbach, B.S.N.,R.N.
Parish Nurse

Article regarding a successful "blood drive" my church set up for me where 40 – 50 people both members and non-members showed up to donate blood, sweat, and time.

TIMES ■ TUESDAY, DECEMBER 5, 2000 **3A**

MEDICINE

a drug hailed
eakthrough'

product of an abnormal chromosome, leads to a huge increase in the number of white blood cells in the body, which can interfere with the functioning of other organs.

Glivec blocks a signal that protein sends out and effectively prevents the abnormal growth and production of other cancerous cells.

"The whole of cancer research has been to identify the differences between cancer cells and normal cells. That's been the goal of cancer research and here it is," said Brian Druker, an Oregon Health Sciences University researcher who was the drug's principal developer. "I view it as a new era of cancer therapeutics. It's the most effective treatment we know of for CML."

Researchers chose CML because they knew about the abnormal chromosome and its abnormal protein. They are hoping to transfer the model — targeting a specific abnormality with minimal effect on healthy tissue — to other cancers, but first they must isolate those cancers' causes.

Currently, bone marrow transplants are the only proven way of curing leukemia, but the transplants carry a mortality rate of up to 40 percent and are only successful in 55 to 65 percent of cases. Other drugs are used to maintain the health of leukemia patients but don't decrease the number of white blood cells or help make the blood normal again.

Glivec has been studied on humans for only about two years, so how long it will prolong a patient's life is not yet known. But it has had few side effects, and only about 2 percent of patients stopped using it because of those side effects.

The drug is expected to hit the market in June. In the meantime, patients who hope to receive the treatment have to join a clinical trial.

Another article on the break-through treatment for CML.

Underlined portion reads: "...currently, bone marrow transplants are the only proven way of curing leukemia...", and the annotated portion, "...not necessary for Ryan – Thank goodness!..."

The irony of this is not lost, as bone marrow transplant was very necessary for me...!

1-11-01

Dear Woelfel Family:

My sincere thanks to your entire family for coming to spend time with us during the blood drive on Saturday!

Ryan and your beautiful wife showed so much courage in your conversation. After all, it's your _dream_ life that is being tested.

Lou, I keep thinking of you and your love for your brother. You certainly must be commended for your unselfish gift of love.

Glen & Patti - for you I saw a deep rooted faith in you as you witnessed in Bible Class comments. Now God is testing you as you have never been tested befor. However, with God nothing is impossible. He Himself commands: "Call upon me in the day of trouble I will deliver thee, and thou shalt glorify me." I am praying and thinking of you all the time.

In Christian Love,

Just Leona Kobel

CHAPTER 5: TRANSPLANT

It was January 27th, we were headed up to begin the admittance process and chemo would start the next day, but first on the schedule was one more biopsy to make sure I was still in remission. I thought my first biopsies went well, procedurally speaking, until Dr. Rosenfeld performed one. Aside from my "youthful" hard bones, bending the needle, and Dr. Rosenfeld having to pull with enough force to pull me off the table, the procedure went relatively well. Dr. Rosenfeld was real into research and statistics, so much so my mom felt he would not have taken my case, if he didn't think I had a strong chance of survival – I guess a 65% chance was considered strong. Dr. Rosenfeld was a true research scientist, who was very proactive and didn't want to wait on pathologist review of my bone marrow biopsy, so he looked at it himself under the microscope. We later learned because of what he noticed while doing the biopsy, why he wanted to personally review the slides. He mentioned I had what he called a "white out," which basically means he was concerned about my disease status. Turns out time was on our side, but just barely, as he said per my bone marrow, I was already in early relapse after completing therapy just a little over two months ago. This revelation confirmed we made the right decision with getting the transplant.

Soon morning arrived with a knock on the door and a nurse was ready to wheel me down to get my first dose of radiation. This was by far the most interesting aspect of my therapy. I was wheeled into a large room with a lot of machines and big thick heavy doors. I had to strip down to nothing and was packed in "long grain" rice. The rice was used to help ensure the radiation would be delivered in a uniform dose across my whole body, as the rice packed around me would make me appear to be one large rectangle to the machine delivering the radiation. I would lay on one side for approximately 30 minutes, then roll over to the other side for another 30 minutes. I was literally like a big meal being microwaved and rotated once, half way through cooking. In fact, this is exactly what was happening, as the radiation waves used in microwaves to cook food, are similar to those used to treat cancer, only at a much lower frequency. I remember contemplating this as I began getting warmer and warmer during my radiation treatment.

With radiation dose one of nine completed, I returned to my room and quickly noticed my skin looked like I had been vacationing in Mexico, but without the sunscreen. It was becoming apparent this round of treatment would be much worse than my prior induction chemo, as I was already experiencing side effects – in walks nausea and vomiting. Keep in mind, this was after only the first round of radiation, of which I would be receiving two per day, and prior to any chemo as well, which would start prior to my evening dose of radiation. This routine of radiation in the a.m. followed by chemo, and then another round of radiation in the p.m. would continue with me eventually receiving nine fractions, or doses, of radiation given over the course of five days, with chemo completing by day three, or d-3 with day zero (d0) being transplant day.

This might be a good time to interject and explain the numbering of the days. Day 0 is referred to as the day the donor cells are infused into the recipient. Anything prior to day 0 (d0), such as conditioning chemo treatment was signified with a d-8, all the way through d0, when the transplant occurs. Everything after d0 is "post" transplant, so it's simply annotated as d1, d2, etc., for day 1 and 2 post-transplant, respectively. Around d-3, so two days after chemo had completed, I began to feel the real effects of this treatment regimen.

My upper GI tract had literally been fried, rather microwaved. I was in more pain than I had ever experienced or thought I would ever have to experience. My mouth was literally raw, and my tongue was swollen about 3 inches thick and looked like ground beef. The pain was excruciating and I was barely able to eat solid foods, and eventually had to be fed through a tube. Never in my wildest imagination did I think drinking water could ever hurt, but my intake was reduced to drinking a drop at a time through a medicine dropper with each drop hurting more than the one before.

This pain was the result of what's called mucositis, which is a side effect of the radiation, and Dr. Rosenfeld said it was the worst he had ever seen in his 20+ years of practice. To make things worse and even more uncomfortable, my body was producing a great deal of mucus to aid in the healing process of the tissue that was damaged through radiation and chemo. Anyone who's ever had mucus knows how uncomfortable it can be, only this was no ordinary case of congestion.

Due to the volume of mucus and my level of pain, I wasn't able to simply cough and spit out the mucus. I had to use a "yankauer," which is a large tube connected to suction in the wall used to vacuum mucus out while at the same time trying not to touch the swollen and fried tissue that had previously been my mouth.

To combat the pain I was in, I was on Morphine and a Fentanyl patch, which are both strong narcotics, but I was still having breakthrough pain. I began to realize just how much of a cake walk induction chemo was for me, as conditioning chemo and radiation were kicking my ass. I was having uncontrolled diarrhea, so bad my ass looked much like my mouth – red, raw, swollen. I was having uncontrolled nausea and vomiting as well, despite the Zofran (antinausea), and Ativan (antinausea, antianxiety, sleep aid). The pain I was in was the worse I had ever experienced. My whole GI tract felt like someone took a branding iron shaped like a rake and scrapped it along my insides. The only time I wasn't in pain, was when I was sleeping. The pain meds were helping, but mostly they would just make me sleep and by the time they wore off, the pain was back and I needed more.

This vicious cycle went on for a few more days, when I abruptly swore off all pain meds other than Tylenol from that point forward. Day 9 post-transplant was the single most defining moment in my transplant experience. Although Dr. Rosenfeld told me I wouldn't remember that day, I remember it like it was yesterday. I went through my normal routine that day, and during the evening, Elisse and I were watching TV, probably "Survivor," as that was the first season and we were intrigued and addicted to watching. I was getting tired and it was time for me to get some sleep. I called in the nurse to request some Ativan, Ambien, and a dose of Morphine, which I was all due for at that time. I took my meds and slept pretty soundly until around 4 a.m. when I awoke in more pain. I called the nurse and asked if it was possible to get more of the same meds I had taken earlier that evening to help me sleep, along with some orange sherbet ice cream. The cold soothed my mouth and throat. After eating my ice cream and taking my meds, I soon fell asleep, and that was the last thing I remember until I abruptly woke up – my whole world turned upside down yet again.

When I awoke from what I thought was a nice slumber, I was standing on my knees in my bed, buck naked covered in blood, shit, piss, and vomit. In my room was an ER doctor, multiple nurses, my wife, security guards, what appeared to be my grandparents from San Antonio, and other people I had never seen before. Out of nowhere I heard "bag him" from one of the doctors in the room. The words that were spoken were in fact the words I had heard; however, the intention was quite different and it depended on which side of the hospital you were on, patient vs. clinician.

Apparently at some point after eating my ice-cream and taking my meds, I had gone into pulmonary arrest. Essentially, I had stopped breathing. This was due in part to overmedication coupled with the amount of mucus I was producing as a result of the profound mucositis I had. I was fading in and out of consciousness and everything was very hazy and ethereal (to use a "Dean Koontz" word). To me, the patient and avid ER watcher, "bag him" was another way of saying "he's done ... put him in a body bag." Immediately my survival instinct kicked in and that was the last thing I was willing to let happen to me. I was determined to show everyone in the room I was far from "done" and in fact, I was very much alive. Now keep in mind that I had stopped breathing, was fading in and out of consciousness, very weak, and on a great deal of pain meds, so my strength would fade in and out and come in bursts of pure energy fueled by the Narcan used to revive me, and then quickly fade to nothing again before I would lose consciousness again.

With these sudden bursts of energy and strength, I would rise up and grab my IV pole and throw it at the docs, nurses, and anyone I thought was trying to put me in a f'ing body bag. I grabbed my tunneled central line catheter – that had been sewed under my skin, hence the term tunneled, and ripped it from my chest leaving scars I still bear today. I grabbed my IV tubing in both hands and snapped it in two, and then all the energy left and I crashed to the bed exhausted and unconscious again. During these times of unconsciousness, I encountered some of the most memorable, scary, and clear experiences I had ever experienced. I'm not sure if what I experienced was what some would call "near death," although, I had in fact stopped breathing and was nearly dead. There was no white light, no calm feeling of peace, yet the amount of clarity I had in those moments I had never experienced prior, nor since. It was as if I was in my own little place surrounded by chaos, outside of what I was experiencing in those moments of unconscious profound clarity. I was surrounded by total complete darkness and overcome with a great deal of fear and uncertainty, so much to the point that I knew I did not want to stay wherever I was and I wanted to get back to where I belonged.

Religion or no religion, faith or no faith your beliefs are your beliefs, and I feel religion is a personal journey left for only one to judge, and it doesn't really matter to me what side you're on. For me, I grew up going to church – Lutheran (as my wife says "twice the 'fun'; half the guilt" – she's a convert). I was active in the church growing up, went pretty much every Sunday, but I wouldn't label myself as overly religious. I have always had a relationship with God, but it's a personal one and I don't force my beliefs on anyone.

During these states of unconsciousness, I felt I was connected here, yet also in this other place simultaneously and in this other place, I only knew I didn't belong – it wasn't hell, but it certainly wasn't heaven; although I had the overwhelming feeling, urge of what I had to do – no, what I needed to do – confess/profess/ testify my beliefs. I heard a voice – it was mine – but not me speaking and I was told if I wanted to get back, I had to testify I needed Jesus and without question that's exactly what I did. As I was coming to and regaining consciousness, I would yell as loud as I could, "I need Jesus...Jesus...I need Jesus!" over and over, all the while, still attempting to keep the doctors, nurses, security guards, etc. at bay with my IV pole. I can only imagine what was going through their minds at this time, and then I heard the doctor say, "He's delirious...he's gonna go under again... bag him...bag him!," and I was off and unconscious again to repeat this cycle. This continued again and again until I saw and heard the one thing that could hold my focus, keep me calm – Elisse.

As I began to regain consciousness yet again, I heard and saw Elisse in the midst of all the people in my room and it was as if, like in the movies, all other sound and periphery ceased and all I could see and hear was her. As she became clearer and clearer to me, I could hear her tell me to calm down, relax, and stop fighting the doctors, they were trying to help me. Seeing her in that instant, I knew I was safe and all was going to be okay and I began to relax and was able to understand the doctors as they explained what had happened to me.

In addition to the calming effect Elisse had on me, she also knew what I liked to listen to and told the doctors to put on some Marty Robbins (I had a "classic country" CD up there with me), to help relax and calm me. As the CD was playing, "The Hanging Tree" started playing. I focused on that song and it was as if the words were speaking to me. Hearing those words and the sound of Elisse's voice combined with the site of her presence, allowed me to stay focused on staying conscious, as I did not want to slip back to the place where I was previously.

At around 6:30 a.m., Dr. Rosenfeld arrived, and I began to piece together what had happened. Due to the severe pain I was in, I had requested more pain meds which I needed for the breakthrough pain I was experiencing. The pain I was in was due to the mucositis I was experiencing from the chemo and radiation, and the amount of pain meds I was on compounded the problem.

I was too sedated to consciously and/or subconsciously realize I needed to roll over and expel the mucus that was blocking my already compromised airway. I was choking on my own mucus and would have died had it not been for Elisse. She woke up to what she thought was me snoring, but she quickly realized I was actually choking, unable to breathe, and unresponsive. When she wasn't able to wake me up, she quickly pushed the call button for the nurse. When my nurse, Mel, arrived in my room, he immediately realized how dire my condition was and began saying, "Call a Code Blue! Code Blue! Code Blue!" Besides me, Elisse was the only other person in the room, so she thought Mel was telling her to call the code blue, to which she responded, "I don't know how to call a code blue? Stop telling me that!" Later she realized Mel was advising the nurse at the desk to call the "code blue" which was the code to get the "crash cart" and rapid response team. Though at the time, none of this was funny, later that day, we were able to laugh about it.

Soon after the code blue was called, my room was immediately filled with doctors and nurses attempting to revive me. I was given three shots of Narcan which is a drug given to people who have overdosed. This drug basically flushes the body of everything, hence the reason I awoke so abruptly finding myself not only confused, but completely naked, wearing nothing but pungent biohazard. Since my cloths had been "biohazarded," they had to be cut from me and disposed of as such. As soon as the emergency response team arrived, they told the floor nurse to get Elisse out of the room. One of the floor nurses, Lourdes, escorted Elisse to the waiting room and advised her to pray.

As I was regaining consciousness, the doctor said "bag him" meaning give me a pump or squeeze of oxygen, clearly not the interpretation I received. They rushed Elisse back in to help relax and calm me down when I started coming to and began having longer periods of consciousness. After Dr. Rosenfeld explained everything to us, he told me I was very lucky, and I had scared him, as his patients usually do not code so early in transplant. I was not exactly comforted and a little confused on how to take his comment "so early." He also told me I would forget the whole ordeal by day's end – clearly not the case, as I write this today. From that moment on, I swore off all pain meds other than Tylenol and Advil.

As the day went on, I did a great deal of reflecting, even more so than I already had since being diagnosed, as that's all there really is to do when confined to a hospital room. I made a decision that I would be out in time for my birthday so I could spend it at home with my family and although that was only three weeks away, I was determined and nothing would stop me.

The remaining days and nights were extremely difficult as the pain was almost unbearable. I was no longer able to eat and had to be fed through my new central line which replaced the one I had ripped out. Due to the swelling from the mucositis, I wasn't able to talk in a fashion where anyone could understand me, which only added to the frustration I was already experiencing with being crammed in a hospital room staring at the same four walls now for three weeks and counting. I had to use a note pad to communicate and was constantly using my suction tube to remove the never-ending mucus. I remember as Valentine's was nearing, this method of communication proved difficult as I was attempting to order Elisse one of those "Vermont Teddy Bears." I had to communicate via my notepad and have my sister, donor, lifesaver, and now secretary, relay this information and be the go between for me and the lady on the phone taking the order. Thankfully it all came together and we were able to get it delivered to Elisse's office without her having a clue.

Being able to do something like ordering Elisse's Valentine's gift helped me feel I was less tied to my condition. Small glimmers of normalcy helped take my focus off all the negative, which is crucial in going through something as serious and scary as transplant. I'm not a negative person, and never once did I wonder "Why me?," but there are good days and bad days and at the beginning, a great deal more bad than good. A crucial part of the recovery process and getting through the bad was the exceptional care provided by the nurses. From making me smoothies to rubbing cream on my ass, no task was too great or small for the nurses and I was, and am, eternally grateful for the care and compassion they gave me.

Together with having great nurses to help get me through transplant, I was also fortunate to have a strong family support system. My sister – not only did Lori provide me w~~i~~ marrow, but she also stayed a long time to assist w whenever she was needed, providing both moral sup ...~~ll~~ as financial. My parents – they were always there to play games, watch TV, talk, or even to apply ointment. I also have to mention my in-laws – they too were great in the ointment application as well, although it was limited to only my feet, which I could definitely understand and respect and appreciate. A big part of getting through this was mental, and this support system greatly helped me remain grounded and maintain a positive attitude.

Another huge part of my support staff, I'm sure unbeknownst to her, was a little girl named Taylor. Taylor was a Godsend in helping me through my transplant journey. She was the only pediatric patient on the transplant floor and her room was next to mine. She was just three years old at the time, and it was her second transplant. She shortly relapsed after her first. I couldn't believe, nor could I even begin to remotely understand how someone so innocent and young and naïve, could have the strength, stamina, perseverance, maturity, willingness, and faith to go through this. I will never forget her and she will always hold a special place in my heart. To this day I often think of her and her family and I still have the "birthday" card she wrote and handed me on my transplant birthday. No matter how miserable I was, I always knew that innocent little girl was going through this as well and her resilience and chipper attitude were a constant reminder that I could come through this as well.

At this point in my hospital stay, my 25th birthday was right around the corner, and although, initially I was sure I would be out in time to celebrate at home, it was becoming pretty apparent this was not going to happen. I developed a condition called veno occlusive disease, or VOD. My liver was starting to malfunction. The indicator for this is a lab value which measures total bilirubin. A high normal is 1.3 mg/dL and mine was at 12mg/dL. This damage was in part due to the toxicity associated with the treatment I had undergone, as well as the heavy drinking I had done in college. Now that my liver was shutting down, that meant I had to stop taking Tylenol. My only options for pain management now were Advil and very limited minor doses of narcotics, as I didn't want to take a chance on coding again.

I felt and looked pretty crummy at this point, especially with the new yellow tone to my skin and eyes and it was questionable as to if I would make it or not. To that point, after I was out of the hospital, Elisse's father told her that after one of his visits to the hospital, he was sure I was not going to make it out of the hospital alive.

Eventually my liver function returned to normal and it was now the day before my birthday. I was happy I was able to see another birthday, but still a little upset I was still in the hospital now going on four weeks with no hope of discharge anytime soon. I was still being fed through a tube, I wasn't able to drink and I wasn't getting out of bed all that much, which were all things that would have to change in order for me to get discharged home. As I dozed off that night, I was slowly beginning to process all of this and understood what it was I needed to do to get out of the hospital.

Morning came and I abruptly woke Elisse up with a loud inaudible yell, when in absolute horror, I sat up in bed at 4 a.m. and hit my face on something dangling from the ceiling. While I was sleeping, Elisse had hung "happy birthday" decorations directly above my bed and when I awoke they were not the fun surprise she had thought they would be. Normally this wouldn't have been a big deal to me, but I was still experiencing some of the after-effects of the pain meds and was literally losing my mind with the lines between reality and fiction constantly blurring.

For many reasons, that birthday was one I will never forget. Elisse gave me a 3-disc CD changer, and a Jim Croce CD. The CD was special because I wanted to play and dedicate "Time In a Bottle" to Elisse at our wedding. While at Tech, before I even met Elisse, this song came on the radio, and after hearing the lyrics, I pulled out a pen and paper and wrote them down.

Whomever, she may be, I knew at that moment, I wanted to dedicate those words to my wife, at our wedding; however, because of my diagnosis, I never got a chance to and this seemed to be Elisse's way of making up for that. Another special gift Elisse got was tickets for us to see David Copperfield which gave me something else to look forward to, a new date to shoot for to get out of the hospital to make sure we could go. I remember her telling me how expensive they were and how they were non-refundable, so I had no choice but to get out. Although, at the time I couldn't see it and even now looking back, I can't see how, but four days later I was discharged and it was the best feeling ever – or so I thought.

Being at home, on our own, away from the nurses, physicians, monitors, and emergency response at the push of a button, was very unsettling. Remember less than three weeks ago, I went to sleep and had coded, so it was extremely difficult to sleep. Additionally, I was still having a hard time with defining the line between reality and fiction, as I was still having extremely vivid dreams still from the effects from all the pain meds I had been on.

Looking back on it now, those instances that balanced somewhere between fiction and reality were some of the most interesting aspects of my experience, though at the time they were some of the most unsettling and frightening.

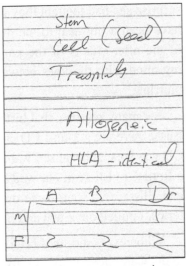

Notes from bone marrow transplantation consult detailing a very simplistic look at HLA typing. Group of 3 (HLA-A, HLA-B, HLA-DR) from Mom and one group of 3 from Dad resulting in 6 that had to match my sister or someone unrelated if she wasn't a match.

...until you're
feeling well again
and always
stay that way.

Will you ever be able to eat rice again after this? Mark loves rice so much he would probably be eating it out of the bag during treatments! 'Course then he would probably begin to glow in the dark. Might be interesting...
God bless and keep you.
Much love from all of us —
The Younger Wolves

Comment asking if I'll ever be able to eat rice again, regarding me having to be packed in rice for the radiation to be delivered at a uniform dose.

Ryan can get **very**
SICK
from our Germs!!!
Please wash your hands when you come in the room! Thanks!

More of Elisse's creativity and artwork

Ryan <u>Woelfel's</u> <u>Room</u>
Please come in if you are here to see Ryan! If not, please pray for him!

Elisse's creativity and artwork

The Texas Cancer Center
at Medical City Dallas

Radiation Oncology

May 25, 2001

Craig S. Rosenfeld, MD
7777 Forest Lane, D-400
Dallas, Texas 75230

RE: Woelfel, Ryan
       50093

Dear Craig:

Ryan completed his total body irradiation as per protocol on 02/02/01. He received a total dose of 13.5 Gy delivered in nine fractions, from 01/29/01 through 02/02/01. B.i.d. fractionation with low-dose distribution for the TBI was utilized.

Overall he tolerated his therapy well and hopefully has had a sustained response.

Again, I thank you for the patient referral and the opportunity to continue to share in his management.

Sincerely,

Louis L. Munoz, MD

LLM/ndb   D: 05/25/01   T: 05/29/01

Total Body Irradiation complete at 1350Cgy over 9 fractions

Dear Woelful Family,

Just a note to say our family is praying for yours. You and your family offer strength with your determination. May God ease your fears and pain in the days to come. Best wishes and may God bless you!

Sincerely,
The Moore Family
Tony, Kim, Kristin & Tis.

Support from my Mom's co-workers

Dear Ryan —

Just got the E-Mails from your Mom & Lori and we are sharing them with your friends here and giving them your new Room #.

We pray all is doing well for you & Lori.

If there is something we can do for you & your family let us know.

May God send complete health to you soon.

Love,
The Halvatsch's
Dennis, Bonnie,
Jessica, Jimmy & Josh

Dear Ryan;

I hear the operation was a success and that you and Lori are on the mend.

Just want you to know that you, Elise, Lori and your Mom & Dad are in our prayers each day.

I know that the Holy Spirit is with you every moment to give you strength and courage and we all await your full recovery soon.

Ray & Marla

Ryan —

We are all pulling for you here at Loguieville. We pray for the best and the quickest recovery.

Love
Andy, Elaine
& Cody

...because that's how much we care.

Dear Elise

We wanted you to know & that we are praying for you. You become a wonderful part of a family and we look forward to meeting you. May God continue to comfort and strengthen you.

we are praying for you

The LORD Helps You

Listen, LORD, as I pray!
    Pay attention when I groan.
You are my King and my God.
Answer my cry for help
    because I pray to you.
Each morning you listen
    to my prayer,
as I bring my requests to you
    and wait for your reply.

    •   •   •

Let all who run to you
for protection
    always sing joyful songs.
Provide shelter for those
who truly love you
    and let them rejoice.
Our LORD, you bless those
    who live right,
and you shield them
    with your kindness.

Psalm 5. 1-3, 11,12

The LORD Is Near to You

Protect me, LORD God!
    I run to you for safety,
and I have said,
    "Only you are my Lord!
Every good thing I have
    is a gift from you."

    •   •   •

You, LORD, are all I want!
You are my choice,
    and you keep me safe.
You make my life pleasant,
    and my future is bright.

I praise you, LORD,
    for being my guide.
Even in the darkest night,
    your teachings fill my mind.
I will always look to you,
as you stand beside me
    and protect me from fear.
With all my heart,
I will celebrate,
    and I can safely rest.

    •   •   •

You have shown me
    the path to life,
and you make me glad
    by being near to me.

Psalm 16.1,2, 5-9, 11a

The LORD Keeps You Safe

You, LORD, are the light
    that keeps me safe.
I am not afraid of anyone.
You protect me,
    and I have no fears.

    •   •   •

I ask only one thing, LORD:
Let me live in your house
    every day of my life
to see how wonderful you are
    and to pray in your temple.

In times of trouble,
    you will protect me.
You will hide me in your tent
and keep me safe
    on top of a mighty rock.

    •   •   •

Trust the LORD!
Be brave and strong
    and trust the LORD.

Psalm 27.1,4,5,14

The LORD Loves You

Your love is faithful, LORD,
and even the clouds in the sky
    can depend on you.
Your decisions are always fair.
They are firm like mountains,
    deep like the sea,
and all people and animals
    are under your care.

Your love is a treasure,
and everyone finds shelter
    in the shadow of your wings.
You give your guests a feast
    in your house,
and you serve a tasty drink
    that flows like a river.
The life-giving fountain
    belongs to you,
and your light gives light
    to each of us.

Our LORD, keep showing love
    to everyone who knows you,
and use your power to save all
    whose thoughts please you.

Psalm 36.5-10

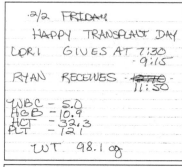

```
·2/2 FRIDAY
HAPPY TRANSPLANT DAY
LORI    GIVES AT 7:30
                   - 9:15
RYAN RECEIVES - ~~7:30~~
                   11:50
WBC - 5.0
HGB - 10.9
HCT - 32.3
PLT - 121
    WT  98.1 og
```

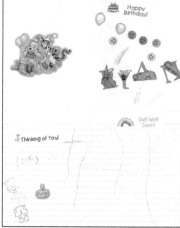

Transplant Day – Day (0) – Lori had almost 3 litters of bone marrow harvested from her and a few hours later it was transplanted into me in a bag similar to a blood transfusion.

> Dear Ryan,
>
> Here's hoping the days will pass quickly
> until you feel well once again.
> Remember that warm thoughts and wishes
> are with you each day until then.
> We just wanted you to know that we are thinking of you daily. You and Elisse are in our hearts and prayers. We pray that this illness will soon be behind you and many happy times together ahead. Love, Kathi & Larry

Supportive card from Elisse's Aunt and Uncle

Hope you enjoy the photos! The girls remember you in their prayers every night. Margi is the "Star of the Week" in her class (they each get "their" week). We worked on a poster and she wanted a photo of the wedding that showed her in her flowergirl dress. She explained that you were bald because you were sick and had to take special medicine that made your hair fall out. I thought that was pretty darned good for a 6 year old. She also has photos of the beach and when she was a baby and when she and Elissa played dress-up one day.

We sure hope you are doing better soon, Ryan. We love you dearly.

God bless and keep you in His abiding presence.

Love,
Mark, Kim, Margi, & Elissa

The 3 year old in the room next to me, Taylor, was also undergoing a bone marrow transplant, but this was her 2nd one at the time. I remember she came in to my room and gave me this card she made for me for my "transplant birthday" – the strength, courage, and determination she had was a definite driving force in my will to survive. I will never forget Taylor and know one day we will meet again in the next phase of life.

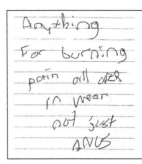

One of the notes I had to write because talking hurt too much. Here I'm asking for anything for the burning pain I was feeling all over my GI tract.

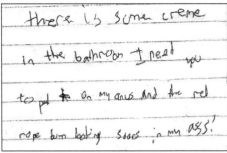

I needed someone to wipe cream on the "red rope-burn looking sores" on my ass!

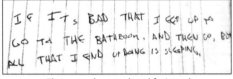

Flat out exhausted and fatigued

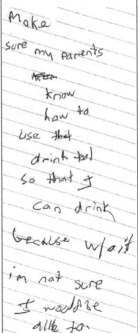

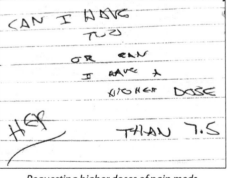

Requesting higher doses of pain meds

I asked if my parents knew how to use the "drink tool," which was a medicine dropper I was using to drink 1 drop at a time due to the pain from the mucositis that resulted from the chemo and radiation.

Tuesday, February 6

Dear Ryan,

We were so glad to hear that the transplant went well! We hope that all of this will be behind you soon. You continue to be in our thoughts and prayers. Get Well Soon.

Cadmus and Sharon Brown

2/8 - THURSDAY   DAY +5

WBC - 0.1
HGB - 12.2
HCT - 36.4
PLT - 8

Stopped breathing momentarily about 5:10 a.m.

over-medicated - gave him something to bring out drugs & he lost control, started fighting - pulled out port

On top of his bed fighting off my ER doctors! Pulled out the port

Temp. 37.9   100.1

Journal entry – stopped breathing/ over medicated. Fought ER docs. Pulled out port.

HOW LONG HAVE I BEEN SLEEPING?
JUST ABOUT 15 MINS?

COME CHECK ON

ME FREQUENTLY

TO MAKE SURE

After coding, I was terrified of sleeping, because I wasn't sure if I would wake up again, or where I would wake up. I was requesting to be frequently checked on.

Dear Ryan —

We've been receiving Lori's E-Mails and it sounds like you have been through hell + back (litterally). Please know that you are in our prayers continually.

You're special in a way no one else is...

I truly believe God won't take you yet, because he has plans for you. You will come out of this stronger + have such a willing + peaceful heart for Him.

So, get lots of rest, grow stronger, and remember you're thought of fondly.

Hope you're Better Real Soon!

We love you

Dennis, Brusie Jessica, Jeremy + Joshua

Howdy folks

As of today, he's doing okay. That's if you take into consideration all the pain he's in from the radiation, and he doesn't really want to take too much pain medicine anymore, and he's not getting a whole lot of sleep. His counts are still very low (expected), he's getting platelet transfusions (blood transfusions on the way), and we're just sitting around waiting until the bone marrow starts to work on him. He does have a few new blood cells, which means something's happening.

Please keep him in your prayers.

-Lori
(more detailed stuff below, if you want to read it)

Here's the gross part. Please don't feel obligated to read this. (Sorry if I caught you while you're eating).

According to him, and the nurses, his mouth and throat look and feel like some madman took a razor blade and cut out a good chunk of stuff, all the way down to his stomach. And his face, throat, and mouth are all swollen as well. Because of the pain he was in, last week he was taking a ton of medicine (morphine is the only med I remember, but I don't know half the names they're calling it). One of the medicines he has been taking for anti-rejection causes him to have mucusitis (very fun to listen to and watch).

On Thursday morning, he stopped breathing. They're thinking now it's because his tongue was swollen, the mucus wasn't letting him breathe too well, and he had a lot of drugs in him. Anyway, luckily Elisse (his wife) woke up to her alarm (she gets up at 5:00 am – how she does it, I don't know). She heard him making a gurgling sound. Thinking it was hiccups again, she tried talking to him. He didn't answer so she called the nurse in. He did the respiratory CPR on him, called a CODE BLUE, and all these ER guys rushed in. They gave him this medicine to take out ALL the drugs in his system (through every orifice you can think of). Elisse was watching this whole thing, and it wasn't fun.

Ryan was in hell. The doctors were going to give up on him. He wasn't going to let that happen. He kept hearing phrases like "bag him," "he's losing it," etc. He most definitely wasn't going to give up that easily. He started fighting for his life. He was asking God for forgiveness, and trying to find out what he'd done that was so bad to end up in this hell. As answers to the doctor's questions, he was saying "No, God is going to save me," "I'm not ready to die yet," but they weren't listening. He yelled a little bit louder, thinking they weren't hearing him.

It took 4-5 people to hold him down. He had kicked the IV pole down, ripped out his IV port (from the muscle in his shoulder which goes to that big vein), and wasn't going to let the doctors give up on him. He was fighting for his life, but the doctors were too. They like Ryan, they're not going to get rid of him that easily. It took Elisse to calm him down. He started recognizing people (Elisse, his nurse, the doctor who put in the first port – who just happened to be on the floor at the time, and came into the room to put the second one in.

Needless to say, he's a little scared to sleep right now, but he's getting better (and so is Elisse). He's always hooked up to an oxygen monitor to keep an eye on him, and he's sleeping with oxygen every night. It's still very painful to eat or drink, but that should clear up in a couple of days, along with the mucusitis. (He's constantly using this dental suction thingy to clear out his throat).

As the doctor said, "It was a scary thing, but not dangerous."

Please keep praying for him. God won't give us anything that we cannot handle, it just gets a bit rocky at times.

—Lori.

Lori's emails updating people about my recent coding episode

Subj: **Ryan -**
Date: 2/12/01 4:24:25 PM Central Standard Time

Dear Lori,-

Thank you so much for sending me the report
on Ryan. It was bad and scary to hear about him, so
terrible! I know that you, Ryan & Elisse have yet to
get your hearts straight, and I don't think I ever
would! Something like that is - well, its terrible!

I thank you so much and I'll keep my prayers
going.   Always,   Marie -

Subj: **Re: A new week in the life of Ryan**
Date: 2/12/01 3:53:55 PM Central Standard Time

Lori, gee, thanks for all the great details but thank the dear Lord that Ryan fought like hell. We're are saying prayers every
minute of the day for both of you and tell him to hang in there. Big hug from me to both of you.
Anne Winters

Subj: **Re: A new week in the life of Ryan**
Date: 2/12/01 4:06:49 PM Central Standard Time

Lori,

We have been praying for Ryan and your family. This is a difficult situation to bear. However, I know the Lord will not give us
more than we can bear. Keep the faith and tell Ryan to fight this battle---he has too much to live for. His testimony will be
the strength of his for living.

Take care Lori,

Gene Watson

Subj: **Re: A new week in the life of Ryan**
Date: 2/12/01 2:01:30 PM Central Standard Time

Our prayers are with Ryan. Please let him know that many, many people are praying for him, and there is nothing more
powerful than prayer.

Subj: **Re: A new week in the life of Ryan**
Date: 2/12/01 2:01:41 PM Central Standard Time

Ryan:

Our thoughts and prayers are with you.

Lila and Dalton

Subj: **Re: A new week in the life of Ryan**
Date: 2/12/01 3:40:14 PM Central Standard Time

Hey girl,

Was just logging on to send an email to ya. Wanted to ask you if you received the second delivery of mail, and to ask if we
should send more.....but in light of your email about your brother and what he is going through, it just seems tacky to ask
"hey, how long ya gonna be there and do you want us to keep sending your mail?"

So I won't ask that.....just want to say that we are praying for you all and hope Ryan continues to get better. Also, hope you
are doing well too and feeling better from the bone marrow procedure.

Love,
Carole and the boys.

Subj: **Re: A new week in the life of Ryan**
Date: 2/12/01 2:39:06 PM Central Standard Time

Wow! I'm glad everything is under control now.

Subj: **Re: A new week in the life of Ryan**
Date: 2/12/01 12:43:51 PM Central Standard Time

As always, appreciate the update. We really enjoyed our visit and dinner
SAturday night, especially since Glenn paid for everything. I am thinking,
next time it should be Lori since we are all paying taxes that support her
very comfortable living. Ha! Ryan is very lucky as I am sure everyone is
aware of to have such a strong, loving and devoted wife. Have a good week
with no surprises and keep us in touch. You all as always will be in our
daily prayers.

ScriBners

I'm praying for you...
that Jesus will touch your body
and restore you to perfect health.
Even more, though, I'm praying
you'll seek Him
in all of His love and grace
and invite Him into your heart...
where He can give you a healing
that will last forever.

I hope that you like this gift that I have sent you. Most importantly, though, I hope that anytime you begin to feel sick, weak, overwhelmed with pain or ready to give up that the scripture on this gift will motivate and inspire to keep on fighting and never give up. For the first time now after having spoke to your mom recently, I realize how serious this really is and I regret not calling your mom more often and keeping in touch like Bobby has. Just remember, that there isn't anything that cannot be conquered through Christ! In the end, he will always be victorious! Please keep in touch and we all are pulling for you. Talk to you later.

Your Brother in Christ,
Nathan Thurman

Get well soon...
you're in good hands!

We think of you
& your family
daily.
Cheryl & Norice

2/13/01
Hope you are feeling better.
We think about you everyday
& say a prayer.

Sorry to hear you're
not feeling so great.
Just wanted you
to know that
you're being thought of
and wished
a quick recovery.

Love,
Damon, Sandy, Nathan
& Jason

Your Dad told me about
your ordeal. I'm happy it
all turned out good.
    Hang in there it will
all get better.
    We don't know why the
Lord sends us all these
things but like our preacher
always says He sends it for
our very best good
    Nighty Nite
    and I love you.
Give my love to the rest of
the family and happy valentine
to all of them too.

Hey Ryan
You do so many things,
Grandson,
to brighten up the year,
It's nice to send you
lots of love
when special days are here!

Happy
Valentine's Day
Lots of love
Grandma

Thanks for being so wonderful... thanks for just being you!

Happy Valentine's Day

DAD ;n LAW

Thinking of you
while you are ill,
and praying
that you find
comfort in the power
of Christ.

I spoke with your father recently and rejoice with you that you responded so well to the bone marrow test. My prayers are with you. Love—
Leona Kohl

Supportive card from
father-in-law

HEY BUDDY——

I HOPE ALL IS GOING WELL UP THERE. BE A GOOD BOY AND TAKE YOUR MEDICINE! MARGI WANTED TO SEND ALONG SOME HEARTS FOR YOU. SHE'S GETTING INTO PORTRAYING OBJECTS AND—IF YOU ARE A GOOD BOY— SHE MIGHT SEND YOU ONE OF HER FAMOUS "PORTRAITS OF PRODUCE" SERIES. IT'S WORTH WAITING FOR.

TAKE CARE AND HANG IN THERE. MORE GOODIES FORTH COMING. STAY TUNED.

MARK

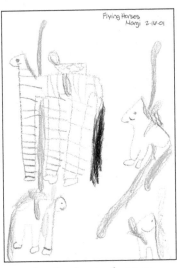

Another drawing from my
2nd youngest cousin – sister to the
youngest cousin

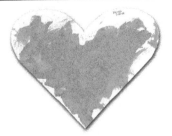

Drawing from my
youngest cousin at the time

2/18   Sunday   Draft 16

WBC   0.1
HGB   8.0
HCT   23.3
PLT   17

Temp ~ 38.6 ↑ 101.5   5 p.m.
BP. 169/100

Ryans feet hurt and his mouth hurts

a Respiratory therapist came in + gave him a toy to increase lung action + coughing so fluid wont settle in his lungs

*He is sucking up some blood from his suction.

Ryan is miserable!

Hopefully WBC will rise tomorrow!

8 p.m. 38.9-102   170/103

Absolutely miserable at this time as the journal entry states. This is also when the lung torturing device was given to me.

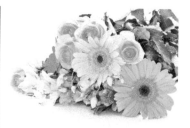

Dear Ryan and Elisse,

Just take
one step
at a time.

We know that there is nothing we can say to make this easier, just know that our thoughts and prayers are with you.

Love,
Daryl
and
Ariana

Supportive card from
Elisse's cousin

This dog is goofy - but it kinda looked like the coopster So we picked this one for you. ☺

You are a toughy to pick something out for- so this book was a recommended read. Hope it might interest you.

I want you to know you are a permanent fixture in my heart and you will be in my prayers throughout this and forever.

you are a strong, strong person and I know you will conquer this.

If ya'll need anything at all- I am readily available - a phone call away.   Take care of yourself - Kelley

Supportive card from Kelley, one of my neighbors in college at Tech. Her co-worker was the first person I shared my experience with as he was newly diagnosed with AML and wanted to hear my story.

Subj: Re: Ryan should be getting out this week
Date: 2/27/01 10:37:44 PM Central Standard Time
From: John & Shirley Vickers

Hi Lori,

   Thank you so much for the update. Elisse said there was a good possibility Ryan would be released sometime this week, so we will keep praying that it becomes a reality soon, and that things just keep getting better and better.

   Love, Shirley & John

Subj: Re: Ryan should be getting out this week
Date: 2/28/01 7:42:56 AM Central Standard Time

Lori, having gone through this in my family recently, I can give great optimism because all things are still working for us. My aunt is in her third year of remission and a professor at AM Kingsville.

I need to talk to your mom. Could you have her call me collect at school. 512-515-6516

I hope you are doing okay. I can only imagine how I would be feeling if my brother, who is my frind too, was going through this. My love to all

Kathy

Well, Ryan missed getting out of the hospital on his birthday (or on Mom's - today), but the doctor did give him a piece of good news. He probably won't have to spend another weekend in the hospital, and the doctor indicated that he might get out Wednesday or Thursday. His counts are going up, we don't have to wear masks (starting today), most of his IV fluids are changing into pill form, and he's trying to eat.

His blood counts are going up considerably, without any help from any white blood cell stimulation medication. He wasn't too happy to spend his 25th b-day in the hospital, but he made it through. Now we're going to sit around and wait until he gets out and take it from there.

He definitely needs your prayers to get through the next few years, trouble free. The next update should come out when he gets home.

Thanks again for all of your thoughts and prayers.

--Lori

Subj: Re: Ryan should be getting out this week
Date: 2/28/01 4:18:26 PM Central Standard Time

Lori we are praying hard for you all. Sounds like things are looking up. Keep us posted on Ryan's progress . We send happy birthday greetings to both your mom and Ryan. Wish we could be there to help out somehow, maybe when things settle down we could make a trip to the ole lone star state, we'll see how things go. You take care of yourself and give all the family our love.
                                                             Jon & Janice

Lifting you up in prayer,
and asking God
to bless you
in many special ways
as you recover.

Ryan, just wanted you to know that we continue to think about you and pray for you. I have lots of time to pray on my commute from Salado to Liberty Hill every morning. My prayer is for you every morning. My prayer is that you will experience complete healing. I also pray for Elisse, Lori, and your mom and dad. I know this has been hard on all of you. Will continue to think about you. Love, Mrs. C.

Supportive card from one of my 6th Grade teachers

Subj: Re: Ryan should be getting out this week
Date: 2/28/01 7:48:01 AM Central Standard Time

Woelfels,
I'm glad things are going well. It's a bummer that Ryan was in the hospital for his birthday, but there will be many more birthdays to celebrate outside. Ryan is in my prayers, and he is in the Hands of the One who has Control.
Love to you all,
Sarah

Subj: Re: Ryan should be getting out this week
Date: 2/28/01 8:26:59 AM Central Standard Time

Praise God! Happy 25th to you Ryan and Patti Happy Birthday to you! I didn't know that Ryan was almost your birthday present. I'm so glad to hear that you guys will be leaving the hospital soon. I know that is really getting old. Beside you are supposed to be on you honeymoon and so far you;ve gotten jipped. We definitely will keep you on our prayer list. Lori, are you recovered? I hope so! You'll take care. lots of love Diane

---

Subj: Re: Ryan should be getting out this week
Date: 2/28/01 8:51:01 AM Central Standard Time

Hooray, Lori and many prayers to you and Ryan and everyone. What an ordeal and hopefully, with God's help the next few years will be good. Good luck and much hope from us. Keep us posted.
Anne Winters

Subj: Ryan
Date: 2/28/01 1:06:09 PM Central Standard Time

Dear Lori,
    I'm so glad that Ryan is doing so well & that he's going home soon! That's the best news!
    I'm glad also, that you don't have to wear those surgical mouth pieces anymore! Every little thing helps, tho I was amazed at Elisse having to wear them all night long!
    Are you going to stay at Ryan's house for the time left? I know you are sick & tired of the hospital! If you can, I hope you come by here and stay for as long as you please! I would love to have you.
    Marie -(Elisse's Grandmommy)

Subj: **Life**
Date: 2/22/01 10:59:36 PM Central Standard Time

Hey Ladies!
I finally talked to my friend, Lisa Uhl, (one of Elissa's godmothers) this evening. She goes out with a guy in Dallas on occasion who is a cancer survivor of about 7 years now - he had APL - a rare form of leukemia. He has been very interested in Ryan's progress and asks for an update whenever he talks to Lisa. He never had a bone marrow transplant and underwent what was at the time experimental treatment but told Lisa he suffered from terrible hallucinations from pain medication. She can't remember which medication caused it - said it had about 15 letters in the name - but said that he thought he was going crazy for awhile. Just thought you might want to know.
Granny called to say that she had talked to Patti and Ryan's numbers were beginning to come up. PTL!
Great news! Give him a hug for us.
Love to all, Kim, Mark, Margi, and Elissa

Subj: **in the dark-Amy**
Date: 2/23/01 12:07:39 AM Central Standard Time

Hi. I tried calling you today at your parents house and Mom told me you're at Ryan and Elisse's.

I thought when they got married he was on the road to remission, why the bleep is he still in the hospital?!?!

I DO NOT UNDERSTAND..................................

How are you feeling? Are you sick because of what you contributed to help your brother's fight for his life? I am frustrated and feel helpless and PISSED that the stupid people we trust to take care of us ,and pay to do so , don't know how much fricken medicine to give him and if it wasn't for his wife the first time and his dad the last, he may not even be here!!!!!!!?????????!!!!!!!

Am i understanding all of this correctly???

How long are you staying in Texas? Is work being understanding? Could you give me Ryan and Elisse's address so I can send them a wedding gift.

Any suggestions?

How are you altogether?

hanging in there? Strong on the outside, as always, I am sure:-)

Well I miss you, all of you and I love you more! Write me back please.

Amy

Well girl -- it's been pretty stressful, but we're all surviving. Yea, I'm at Ryan and Elisse's house in Plano, since the 31st of Jan. He was in remission, all the cancer was gone from his body. However, he had a pretty high chance that it would come back in 18 months. Since we didn't want that to happen, and I turned out to be a perfect bone marrow match, he decided on the transplant to have a chance of a little longer than 18 months -- like 90 years or so. That's why he's in the hospital when he wasn't sick, and it really stinks. He's getting really frustrated right about now, but we had him on the Play Station (my friends let him borrow one).

He's still going through all the side effects, not from the transplant, but from the chemo and radiation they had to use on him to kill his current (well, it's not there anymore) bone marrow, and make room for mine. That's what's pumping through him right now, and his blood counts are going up, which means he's almost able to get out of the hospital. We still have around 2 years to go in which to make sure that this transplant worked. After that time, the Doctor says he's pretty much cured.

I'm only sick cause I caught some kind of sinus/throat infection. Not a big deal to me, but since Ryan can't handle any sicknesses now (his immune system is WAY down, but on the way back up), I had to stay home for a while. The Doctor's say everyone is different, which is most likely why they don't know how much meds to give him. He's a big guy, so they've based most of it on that fact, but his medicine reaction doesn't work that way.

I'm gonna stay here until he gets out, and most likely a few weeks afterwards to help out with transporation to/from doctor's offices. Work is being okay so far, but I'm about to run out of leave, so we'll see how long that lasts.

Ryan and Elisse Woelfel

Wedding suggestions: I have no clue. I still need to send Jakey a present. They're registered at Target if that helps.

anyway, I should go to sleep now, it's almost midnight.

I'll talk to you soon. Take care, and keep praying.

--Lori

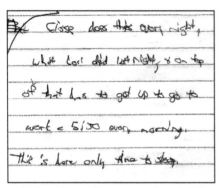

Elisse does this every night, what load did last night, & on top of that has to get up to go to work @ 5:30 every morning. This is here only time to stop.

I'm bragging on how strong, thoughtful, caring, and supportive Elisse is and has been through all this.

9:00p Ryan VERY Dopey looking, esp w/in the last hour. At Ryan's request, Dad removed TS patch. Karen called Rosenfeld to ask to decrease patch

Was beginning to look very "dopey" again, so I asked my dad to pull the fentanyl patch off me, I was using for pain, as I didn't want to code again.

Ryan,

May you look to God our Father with hope and faith and prayer, knowing that He keeps you in His tender, loving care.

Trusting To See You Better Soon

Though the road at times is uphill — there's a thought we'd like to share; We're behind you as you're climbing and we're lifting you in prayer!!! May God grant you His strength and courage as you fight this battle!

Love,
Roger, Doreen
Joshua + Tonya
Woelfel

"...Blessed are all they that put their trust in Him."
PSALM 2:12 KJV

Ryan —
a little bird told us that you lost your pocket cross, and we felt you needed another one — so here it is!
We hope this finds you feeling better — we are still praying for you —
Love + blessings
Granny + Paw Paw

I said a little prayer for you today — because you're someone who means so much to me.

Your mom said your counts are remaining good. For that we are thankful.
Love,
Granny + Paw Paw
Did you get the cross?

Note from my grandparents about the cross I "lost" (flushed down the toilet to save the world) and giving me another one to replace it.

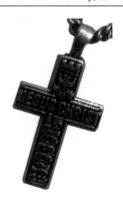

2/25 SUNDAY   DAY +23

WBC- 1.1   SEGS - 69
HGB - 7.6   BANDS - 2
HCT - 22
PLT - 11   ANC - 781

Gets blood & platelets
today

3:30 pm.   4:30 pm.

BP 143/95   Temp. 36.6
PULSE 102   BP 136/98

7 pm.

Temp. 37.8 wa.
BP 143/94   100.1

Smiles, has personality,
+ says he feels
100 times better

Rosenfeld "No more week-
ends in hospital"

*My personality is coming back and will
be getting discharged from the hospital
soon. Doing much better at this time.
Started engrafting the day prior.*

Dear Ryan,

As God takes care of us
through each season of the
year .... so He will take
care of you, Ryan.

May God grant you the
peace that passes all
understanding of knowing
"why"!

Jesus loves you!

Marvin & Peggy Kelm

Praying You're Better Soon

Bobby + Judy were here in the
country over the weekend. Judy
called and said to send you
their love and they are praying
for you. Tell your Mom and
Elisse hi! and we are all
praying for them too. Dad called
last night. Was glad to hear he
got home safe + sound. Love
They that wait upon the Lord
shall renew their strength..."   Grandma
ISAIAH 40:31 KJV

We hope that
you have a day
full of love and
hope. Happy Birthday
Ryan. You along with
Elisse and your family
are constantly in
"I praise Our prayers. We
You
because pray that you
I am
fearfully will truly have a
and
wonderfully good and happy
made;
Your Birthday.
works
are
wonderful,
I know
that
full
well."
PSALM
139:14 NIV

Just take a peek
in the mirror!!

Yes, you!
Happy Birthday!
Love Corey, Lindsey,
and Matthew.

Elissa awakened at 5:15 this morning with a bad dream. We are writing this card and drawing pictures. She is talking about her upcoming birthday party (in July, mind you). She wants both Barbie *and* Veggie Tales platts, forks, & napkins! Oh, and cups. She is having trouble pronouncing her "R's" so I have to listen very carefully. For instance, "Barbie" sounds like "Bobby" and "fork" sounds like, well, we won't go there.

The backyard is slowly taking shape. Mark is slaving away building stone retaining walls in the back. Next comes truckloads of mulch for the play area. Then we get the irrigation system installed and then solid sod. We plan to get some high school kids from church to help with manual labor - sound familiar?

Margi & Elissa   2·24·01

(HER ARTWORK ON BACK)

Find joy in the little things.

Have a

Happy Birthday

Hang in there, cutie! We hope this is the happiest of birthdays for you - we hear you are on the mend and are so very grateful. God bless and keep you in His protective arms. We love you, HANG IN THERE, IT'S ALL DOWN HILL NOW...

Psalm 4:7-8   Mark, Kim, Margi & Elissa

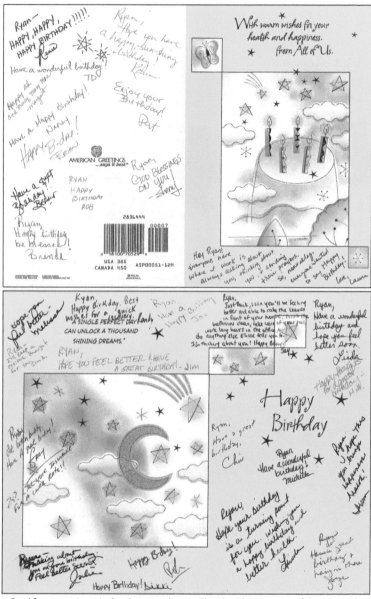

Card from my sister-in-law's co-workers in Florida. I know none of these people, yet they took the time to really write some heartfelt words.

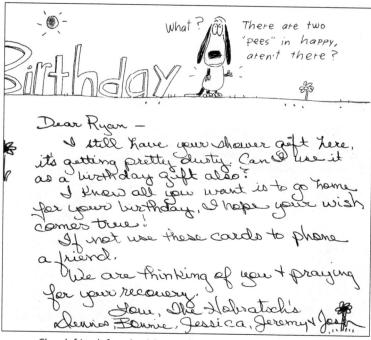

Church friends from back home giving me phone cards I could use
to call people if needed, when I was bored sitting in the hospital.

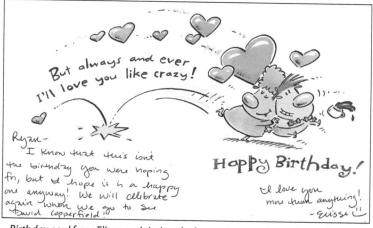

Birthday card from Elisse, exclaiming she knows I was hoping to be out by now,
but we'll just have to plan to be out in time to see David Copperfield.

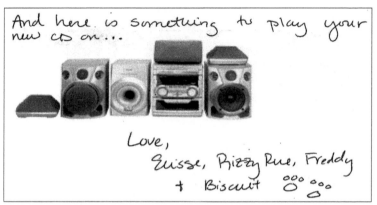

And here is something to play your new cds on...

Love,
Elisse, Rizzy Rue, Freddy
+ Biscuit

New stereo system Elisse got me for my birthday that I could use to play the Jim Croce CD on it that had the song, "Time In A Bottle" on it.

---

*W*ishing you strength
for each tomorrow
through the
love and hope
that surround you
today.

RYAN —
CONGRATS ON THE GOOD NEWS!!
I REALIZE IT WILL BE DIFFICULT FOR YOU
TO LEAVE THE HOSPITAL, BUT I KNOW YOU'LL
MANAGE!! TAKE CARE BUDDY
MARK

3½ FRIDAY   DAY + 28

WBC — 2.8
HGB —
HCT — 26.0
PLT — 36   ANC - 1512

GO HOME TODAY!

IN OFFICE 9 A.M. MONDAY 3/5

Going Home!

Congratulations on those rising numbers! It was so good to hear that you are beginning to feel like yourself again!
God bless you — We love you!
Mark, Kim, Margi, and Elissa

MEDICAL CITY DALLAS HOSPITAL
7777 Forest Lane
Dallas, TX 75230

PATIENT: WOELFEL, RYAN G
PHYSICIAN: Craig S Rosenfeld, MDx
MRN: 000000H000761787
ACCOUNT No.:

DISCHARGE SUMMARY

DATE OF ADMISSION: 01/26/01

DATE OF DISCHARGE: 03/02/01

HOSPITAL COURSE:
This 25-year-old was admitted to undergo allogeneic transplant
for high risk AML and 1CR. He was diagnosed on November 16, 2000.
He had high risk AML based on his cytogenetic findings.

Pretransplant evaluation revealed that he was both in psychologic
and molecular remission.

The patient was admitted to the hospital on 1/26/01. The
preoperative regimen consistent of cyclophosphamide and total
body radiation. Graft versus host disease prophylaxis consisted
of Cyclosporin plus Methotrexate.

The transplant was performed on February 2, 2001. Stem cells were
obtained from the marrow of an HLA identical sister.

Ingraphment was a bit delayed. A neutrophil count greater than
500 was achieved on day 22. During the hospitalization, the
patient received 14 platelet transfusions, and 5 red cell
transfusions.

The major complication was grade 3 stomatitis. The patient
required TPN but not amphotericin. There were no documented
inspections. The patient also developed veno occlusive disease on
day 11. The maximum bilirubin was equal to 9. At the time of
discharge, the bilirubin is approximately 5 and is decreasing.

DISCHARGE MEDICATIONS:
Cyclosporin, Septra DS, Prevacid, and Norvasc.

DISCHARGE INSTRUCTIONS:
Mr. Woelfel will be seen in the transplant office in three days.

Craig S Rosenfeld, MDx

CSR:EDiX11748
D: 03/02/01 10:36 T: 03/06/01 13:16 DOCUMENT: 200103020213997500

Discharge Note from Dr. Rosenfeld, covering my 36 days in the hospital.

CHAPTER 6: CRAZINESS ENSUES

With all the treatment I had undergone, possibly coupled with my liver beginning to shut down, I was literally losing my mind and the line between reality and fiction had disappeared. Here are some of the accounts of those dreams and instances where I hung somewhere in the balance between reality and insanity. Each of these instances described below are those that are most vivid today. These accounts are how they seemed to me at the time they were happening in my head, and seemed as real to me then, as my sitting here writing this today.

House with Nazi Memorabilia and Pornographic Video Games

Elisse and I were living in a house that had four stories. It had a basement and the driveway connected both the basement and the fourth floor – the impossibility of that didn't come into play at the time. The fourth floor was really more of a set of stairs about six or so that went up through a crawl space to enter a room large enough for only a couch, placed under a small window. The third floor consisted of a dark hallway leading to a dark room with a great deal of Nazi memorabilia, including pictures of Hitler, the Nazi flag, etc, and pornographic arcade style video games. The first floor was also dark and had brown shag carpet, two brown recliners, and a long brown couch. The walls were dark wood paneling. I never saw much of the other floors so I can't really describe them, other than I know they were there.

We shared this house with another family I presume, although I only saw and spoke with one other person, a guy in his 50's who only wore "tighty-whities" and a white t-shirt and always had a brown blanket wrapped around him. I can't recall what we talked about, but I remember he, too, was a cancer patient and had been through a similar treatment I had been through, so we talked about that. He also had a couple of dogs (Dachshunds) and they would often jump on my lap when I sat down in the recliner.

The dark hall and the large dark room, full of Nazi memorabilia and pornographic arcade games, gave off an eerie feeling of cool, death, darkness, and misfortune. I'm not sure what the significance of this was, but nonetheless, there I was living among it all.

Meeting with Hospital CEO in My House

Apparently, my imaginary house (the one described above), was a very important "meeting" place, because the CEO of the transplant hospital called me requesting to hold a meeting there with three of his colleagues. He told me their usual meeting place was unavailable and thought my house would be a good substitute. I, of course, asked about a discount with respect to my medical bills with the hospital and he agreed we could work something out, and we began negotiating this over the phone. I cannot recall the final discounted rate we agreed upon, but I believe it was in the ballpark of 20% off. This made me very happy because with Elisse and I just starting our new life together, any financial break was a tremendous help and

I figured it was well worth it since I was providing the much needed venue for his meeting.

Elisse told me I woke her up around 3 a.m. to let her know about this meeting and told her of our discount. She was not as pleased as I had figured, as she was living in reality, and in reality it was 3 a.m. and she had to be at work in three hours.

3000AD – Saving and Leading the World – The Cross

It's in the third millennia and I'm in a tent with hundreds of thousands of people surrounding me, much like the situation described in Exodus regarding Moses. We are the chosen people and I their leader and this is the way it has been now for 300+ years. That is the only back story my mind would give me. Elisse, our kids (although in reality I had no kids at this time), parents, grandparents, wife's parents and grandparents, cousins, aunts and uncles, were all in my immediate circle closest to me in the camp, and we would move only when I got the feeling to do so. Everyone was starving, thirsty, angry, and often times questioning my judgment. Although my being their leader in this capacity was old hat to them (300+ years now) in my perspective at that moment in time, it was all new and I hadn't had a clue as to what I was doing there. Furthermore, I couldn't understand why everyone was coming to me for advice. Who made me king and ruler of all these people? Apparently I did, a long time ago.

So I have to interject a bit here to provide a little more background to this story. The line between reality and fiction had become so blurred; I would often times have to use objects to help me identify which world I was in, much like in the movie "Inception" released in 2010. For me, it was a cross from James Avery given to me by Elisse after I had come through the ordeal of coding, meant to give me solace and comfort in knowing who was in control. How this worked, and I'm not sure how, other than the subconscious mind is extremely powerful, but if I were in a situation in one of these dream states and was unable to tell if it was reality or fiction, when I would look down and didn't see the cross, I knew it was all in my head and not real, because in reality I had the cross, and vice versa, for when I wasn't sure if conversations or experiences I was having were real or not, if I saw the cross, I knew it was, in fact, something real.

So back to the story now – I'm leading all of these people and they are extremely pissed off at me and are beginning to blame me for all of their problems and threats are starting to come upon my family. I was at a loss as to what to do and remember thinking, wondering how I could go back to a time before I was in charge. I started to believe all of the hardships and anguish these people, including my own family, were suffering were because of something I had done along the way, a mistake I had made at some point, although not exactly knowing when, what, or why. Then all of the sudden, it hit me and I began to rationalize that being this far into the future is only the direct result of having successfully come through the transplant I had all those many years ago – thousands of years ago – and for that reason I would have to find some way to get back to a time before. I could then undo all this mess I had somehow caused. I didn't want to go too far back though, because I didn't want to have to go through leukemia and transplant again, in case the result was different. I had to think of a time that was back far enough, but just after transplant, so I wouldn't have to relive it.

I began thinking what's the one thing I had that still tied me to transplant, the one sentinel event in my life, after a millennium had now passed, and there it was – the cross. I believed with every fiber of my being, with 100% conviction, if I were to somehow destroy or get rid of the cross, then that would free me and allow me to start over post-transplant. In effect, it would allow me to correct my mistakes so I could lead these people correctly next time around, while at the same time ensuring I didn't have to repeat transplant – pretty smart thinking if you ask me. I told myself this was the only way and as soon as I realized it – BAM! I was now back in reality, and I knew this of course because l looked across the room and saw my cross, as that was my signal for reality, I knew what I had to do. I got up out of bed – it was late in the evening or early in the morning – I grabbed my cross off my food tray, took it in my hand and began to ponder how I could get rid of it, so my future self could get a second chance. I figured the trash wouldn't work because it could be found, and I couldn't just hide it somewhere for the same reason, so I did the only sensible thing to do. I walked in the bathroom, opened the toilet seat, threw it in the toilet and flushed a few times to ensure I had done the job.

I stood there for a few minutes and then it hit me. What had I just done? What the hell – that was stupid and now what was I going to say happened to my cross when someone asks where it is? I felt like an idiot and went back to bed and figured I'd worry about it later. Morning arrived and sure enough, the first question from my morning nurse was wondering what had happened to my cross. I didn't want to tell her about my craziness, so I just said I wasn't sure and played dumb and said maybe it fell somewhere. That poor nurse felt horrible for me and searched and searched and searched my room, the trash, brought the med tech in to change the sheets, had the floor swept, and so on. I know she personally looked for more than 30 minutes and over the next several days she, along with all of us, continued to do so. I felt pretty bad for her, but now, even more so, after all the searching she had done, there was no way I was going to fess up to my stupidity and confess to what I had done.

The searching continued until she made a comment speculating that perhaps one of the cleaning people had swiped it and that she bet she knew just who did it. I wasn't about to let some poor soul get blamed for stealing a cross from a cancer patient, so I spoke up and mentioned I think I recalled what had happened. I said I now remember I had to get up to go the bathroom in the night and grabbed it off my tray to take it with me and I vaguely remember seeing it in the toilet right after I flushed. I explained I must have dropped it in there without even realizing it, as I was so out of it. Elisse heard this and began asking why would I take the cross to the bathroom in the first place. I just told her I was out of it – who knows. The nurse then called plumbing and they said it was lost and there was nothing they could do to retrieve it, as we were on the twelfth floor. I remember thinking to myself – yes, I had succeeded and my future self would be pleased with his past version.

The very next day, my grandmother sent me a new cross that was identical to the one I had flushed. After we got the cross, Elisse got some packing tape and taped it securely several times around the bed rail to prevent this from happening again. When I was discharged from the hospital I took that cross back to James Avery and bought a chain and had them solder a bail on it and I've worn it around my neck from that day forward and have never taken it off. Crazy thing is, I never once had that dream again; who knows perhaps it really did work. After all, Ryan does mean "chosen one" in some translations – I guess time will tell, about three millennia to be exact.

John Glenn – Astronaut Training

During my hospital stay, as a result of the mucositis and the accumulation of mucus in the airways in my lungs, I had developed atelectasis, which is a collapse of the lung. One of the tools used to get my lung function restored was a "volumetric exerciser," a.k.a a torturing device and anyone who has ever used one can attest to that. The volumetric exerciser was designed to increase the "vital capacity" of my lungs, which is the total volume of air one's lungs can store. Improving my lung function was a crucial means to being discharged from the hospital; however, my motivation was lacking due to the pain involved in using it. My motivation quickly changed when John Glenn stopped by for an unannounced visit. John's "mission" was to discuss astronaut training with me.

I must admit, I felt pretty special this legend took time out of his day to give me a pep talk. He visited me on several occasions, and I remember sitting in some chamber that was supposed to help with the breathing exercises. In this chamber, I would swing on a large swing, similar to those at the "San Francisco Steak House," except without all the people eating steak. It was also hard to determine exactly what John Glenn was saying, as I could only hear tidbits as I would swing back down closer to him, but it was something to the fact that if he, at his age could do it, then I surely could as well. He was always polite, very thoughtful, and patient focused, and then he was gone just as fast as he had appeared.

Toy Alien in My Chest

One morning after eating some cereal in my hospital room, I began feeling a strange pain in my throat and chest. I wasn't able to fully describe it or quite understand what it was until I had noticed a toy alien action figure on my cereal box. I then realized I had swallowed this action figure and now it was stuck in my chest. I began freaking out making unintelligible sounds while trying to explain my predicament to Elisse. I was extremely concerned because of all the problems I was already having with breathing and wasn't quite sure how this action figure was going to be removed. Of course at this point in the transplant, I wasn't able to talk or make any sense and had to use a note pad to communicate, which only added to my anxiety and frustration.

Once Elisse realized what I was trying to tell her, she found it pretty humorous, much to my frustration and dismay, because she knew how big this toy was – about the size of toenail clippers. She tried to explain to me at the time that there was no way I could have swallowed it; but it didn't matter because I knew I had. At my request, she then called the nurse to come in with a flashlight to look just to make sure there was nothing lodged anywhere – this of course was after Elisse had pulled the toy out of the cereal box to show me it was still there, but I still knew and insisted it was in my chest.

What makes this story even crazier is I was never given any cereal, and if I had, it certainly would not have been in a cereal box containing a prize.

Sports Radio Talk Show

Dr. Rosenfeld moonlighted at a radio station as a sports talk show host in his spare time when he wasn't seeing patients, giving talks at various speaking engagements, or working in the lab. Convenient for him, his talk show was set up in the hospital right down the hall from my room. He would discuss all kinds of sports and this particular evening, he invited me to come on his show as a guest. I can't really recall what exactly we talked about, but it was something regarding baseball. Seemed like I was there for about two hours and I remember it seemed perfectly normal for us to be doing this sports radio show right there in the hospital. He was still in his doctor's coat so after the show he could continue making his rounds.

Cloning

Even more so devastating to me than my diagnosis, was learning the possibility of becoming sterile and unable to have children being near 100%. Being diagnosed with cancer was unimaginable, but now I felt I was being robbed of my future, and as a result, I was now possibly robbing Elisse of her future ability to have children as well. Even though I had sperm banked, it still would be difficult, expensive, and uncertain if we would ever be able to have children. Additionally, although I was confident I would come through transplant, there was no way to know how long I would be here in this world, as making it through transplant was only part of it. There was always the possibility of relapse, at least up to two years post-transplant. My biggest concern was what if I didn't make it long term? How could I ensure some part of me lived on if, God forbid, I didn't make it? The answer was easy – I would just clone myself.

Now even in my altered mind, I knew this was an extremely delicate, scientific, and highly complex task I was embarking on. I had taken biology in college and was up on the controversy surrounding cloning, as "Dolly" the sheep was in the news at this time. I believed at some level, maybe cloning had been over complicated and the reason we hadn't made a breakthrough is because nobody was thinking simplistic enough – the scientific community was forgetting the basics. DNA is passed through generation to generation via procreation. Now procreation for me at this point wasn't possible because being connected to an IV pole with 15+ tubes, being full of mucus, being nauseated, and out of my mind doesn't paint the most seductive picture, nor does it provide all that sensual of a mood. This was neither here nor there at this point, as I wasn't trying to conceive a child via mixing my DNA with someone else's; I merely wanted to clone myself. This was easy, because I had an endless supply of DNA and I would just have to procreate with myself, and that's exactly what I did (remember this is in my head, as there was no spillage going on while hospitalized).

After scraping each shot of DNA off the toilet, I placed them in six separate specimen grade vials, that just happened to be in my bathroom, and I capped and closed them. Extremely pleased with my achievement, I took those six vials containing my DNA and gave them to the appropriate scientist to complete the process. Later in my hospital stay, I expressed to Elisse that she needn't worry about the future, as I had created six clones of myself and they would all go on to live should something happen to me. I watched as the first of them were given through adoption to several excited couples and I knew all would work out, for I just increased my chances for survival six fold. Even today when I see someone that resembles myself, I point them out to her and make the remark – "there goes one of the six."

Teleportation

The ability to jump from my bathroom in the hospital, straight to the kitchen in my house was a feat I was able to accomplish many times, not fully understanding how, nor knowing when this would occur. Often times, either day or night, I would get up and go to the bathroom and close the door (perhaps to do some more cloning), and upon opening it up and stepping out, I would enter the kitchen in my house. Of course, once I noticed I was in my kitchen, I knew I needed to get back to my hospital room before people noticed I was missing and began to worry. It was a nice break though to get out of the room no matter how brief my stay was. To get back to my room, I would only have to walk back down the hall from the kitchen and open the door and bam, there was my hospital room right in front of me.

My kitchen wasn't the only place I would end up though. Often times I would wind up in the hospital parking lot with the janitorial staff enjoying some Gatorade on the curb. I would also go into other patients' rooms, either by walking through my bathroom door, or sliding through a seam in the wall. The ability to do this seemed as perfectly normal as anything else and I didn't quite understand how unique this teleportation ability was. My hospital neighbors didn't seem to mind me just appearing in their rooms either. In fact, on a few occasions my neighbors ended up being some old high school acquaintances and it was nice to catch up with them. There also was a family I would often see that lived on the balcony outside my room. They were nice, but didn't say too much, and smiled quite a bit, which I often wondered about since the balcony seemed to be a very small place for a family to be living. But I would always say hi to them as they passed my bed with a bag of groceries they had just picked up at the store. They tended to keep to themselves quite a bit, which is probably why I enjoyed their company so much.

Threesome Proposition

This is probably my most favorite encounter, although it could have been much more enjoyable had it occurred, or at the very least, if I could have imagined it occurred with more vivid details. In any case, one of my favorite nurses who had seen me at my worst, must still have found me irresistible, or at the very least, found Elisse irresistible. I always suspected this was weighing on her mind, as I can imagine how attractive I must have looked connected to an IV pole with numerous IV tubes connected with multiple medications running through me. Not to mention the vomit bucket and portable bedside toilet by my bed, as I'm quite sure those items added to the package. And the mucositis and constant sucking of mucus out of my throat with my suction tube, all added to the irresistibility that oozed from me. I couldn't blame her in the least bit, when she leaned over close to my ear and asked if there was any way I would be interested in having a threesome. I admit I was a little taken back by her request, and figured it was probably against hospital policy, but figured that was on her, (and soon I would be as well). In any case when I mentioned it to Elisse later that evening, she brushed it off and seriously doubted I had heard what I had heard; however, the nurse and I did converse about it for quite a while, and after all, you lose all modesty in the hospital, especially as a cancer patient, so she had seen me in all my GRANDEur, so who's to say for sure?

Discharge

The subject of discharge was quite a heated topic with me and almost violent at times and extremely frustrating. On numerous occasions, Dr. Rosenfeld had said I had met all the milestones thus far, my infections had cleared, my counts had returned to normal and I was ready to be discharged out of the hospital to home. Nurses on the other hand didn't agree and would often second guess this decision. Quite frankly, I was beginning to question who was running the show here, the nurses or the doctor. I know now, and so do they. I'd call the nurse in my room around 3 a.m. and inform her that Dr. Rosenfeld and I had just had a meeting in the parking garage and he informed me to tell the nurses I was good to go. The nurse then had the audacity to doubt what I was saying indicating I must have imagined this because it's 3 a.m. and I'm still on IV antibiotics and my ANC is still too low to be released. Additionally, she mentioned it's highly "off protocol" for the transplant doc to be discussing discharge orders with patients in the parking lot, but she said she would check nonetheless. Perhaps she was just upset that the threesome hadn't occurred yet.

Another occasion occurred and this time we were at some other place in the hospital (perhaps on his sports talk radio show) when again Dr. Rosenfeld mentioned all was good and I was to be discharged and I needed to tell the nurses. In fact, he was a little upset at seeing me because he said I should have already been sent home. I told him I had been trying to tell the nurse that he said I was to be discharged and they kept telling me it was all in my head. Still, he assured me he would talk to them and get it sorted out. Of course when I saw the nurse again, I had told her what the doctor had said and she was still very dismissive. This infuriated me, as I had been cooped up in the hospital room for five weeks now, suffered through my b-day, was going crazy, and had been discharged by the doctor, but this nurse refused to let me go. I grabbed my bed pan and began banging insistently on my bed over and over again demanding the doctor's orders be followed, and I be discharged. This in turn woke Elisse up, wondering what the hell I was banging on stuff so early in the morning for. I then calmly explained to her my frustration with the nurses not listening to me. She then explained to me that it was 3:00 in the morning and Dr. Rosenfeld was asleep in bed and that's exactly what I needed to do. Eventually I realized she and the nurse were probably correct, so I relented a bit and said we would sort it out in the morning during rounding, as I knew now on three separate occasions, he tried to discharge me and we would indeed sort this out – then I went back to sleep.

Certainly, the most memorable, interesting, and frightening experiences were those described above. However, they weren't frightening because of the nature of the dreams or experiences, they were frightening because they were so vivid and real-like. I couldn't tell what was real and what was fiction. There were some occasions when large amounts of time had passed – days – in the "fiction" world, only to have me suddenly be in reality and conclude the past three days were all in my head. It would greatly add to my frustration when I would think I was three or four days closer to discharge, only to learn that only one night had passed, or sometimes only a couple of hours.

The experiences outlined above were only the most vivid and most memorable, as there were many more, but mostly just flashes of happenings that were very nonsensical. Some of these experiences lasted long after my discharge and the blur of reality and fiction was so apparent to me that when I did finally get discharged "for real this time," the first thing I did was unload my shotgun and hide the ammo, for I didn't want to be responsible for doing something out of fear in my fictional world that would have horrible consequences in the real world. Even today ... this far out from transplant, sometimes I wonder – way in the back of my mind – if one day I'll wake up back in my hospital room and the past 16 or so years had all been in my head, like that of a season finale in a soap opera.

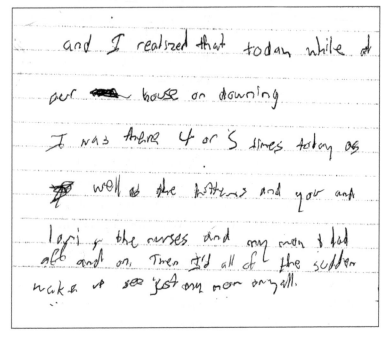

Journal entry about teleportation abilities

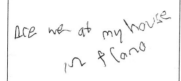

Craziness – wasn't sure if I was in the hospital or at my house or somewhere else.

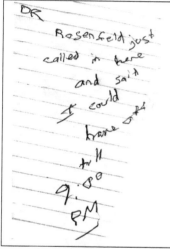

Journal entry regarding Dr. Rosenfeld just discharging me from the hospital to go home, but only until 9:00PM!

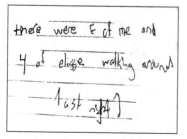

Journal entry regarding my clones walking around

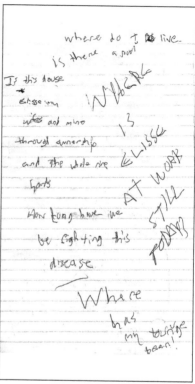

Me quizzing my perception of reality here.

"Is this house Elisse, my wife's and mine, through ownership and the whole nine yards?"

"How long have I been fighting this disease?"

"Where has my tongue been?"

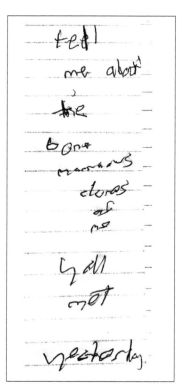

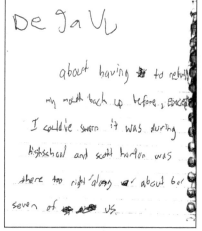

Journal entry regarding having to build up my mouth back up before, but it was in high school and Scott Horton was there along with 6 or 7 other people??

Journal entry requesting my family to tell me about the bone marrow clones of me they got to meet the previous day

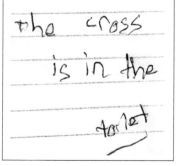

Me confessing where the cross is

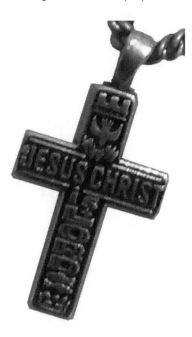

CHAPTER 7: RECOVERY

Getting through transplant wasn't even half the battle, although at the time it seemed I had made it through and it was going to be an easy road ahead. Prior to going through transplant, I was told I could expect to be out of work or on disability for at least six months, at which I scoffed because I knew how strong willed, determined, and tough I was. After all, remember I had youth on my side. Even with the transplant coordinator explaining to me that although I didn't feel like it now, most likely I would come to understand exactly what she was talking about, and boy was she right on the money. My strength and stamina had been severely decreased and I was extremely fatigued. I wasn't able to carry a 20 lb bag of cat food and needed a cart to transport it from the store to my car and had to have Elisse get it out of the car, quite emasculating to say the least. To mow our lawn, which was a normal city sized lot, it took me four hours with having to take breaks every 15 minutes.

Contributing to the difficulty with things getting back to normal was how long it took for my appetite to return. I have always been a big eater, and weighing in at 230 lbs before transplant, it was quite evident. Now, post-transplant, I was at about 170 lbs, and had lost about 60 lbs in about six weeks. The "chemo-radiation-transplant diet," although a highly effective one, I would not recommend it. One of the reasons I lost so much weight, was my body was using every ounce of energy possible to rebuild itself. I was told I needed to be eating at least a 5000 calorie per day diet, to keep up with the energy reserves I needed in order to meet my current dietary needs. Additionally,

I was drinking as many protein drinks as I could stomach and even frequented McDonald's quite a bit, because although the quality was horrible, the quantity was superb for high caloric intake.

On one such occasion, following doctor's orders requesting a high caloric meal at McDonald's, something occurred that will forever be etched in my mind. When I pulled out my cash to pay, the first bill that came out of my wallet had the name "Ashton" written on it in pen. This was a huge deal, as Elisse and I were just talking about and wondering if, and how, we would be able to ever have kids given the near 100 percent certainty of sterility post-transplant. Additionally, even though I had made it through transplant, there was still much uncertainty that lie ahead, as relapse was a possibility at least, up to two years post-transplant, and there was always the possibility of GVHD which could lead to latent organ damage and failure. With all this uncertainty that lie ahead, I had said a prayer asking for a sign, as most of us always do at some point in our lives, a sign everything would be alright and I would come through this and be able to live a normal happy life with a family complete with children.

Months prior to being diagnosed, while we were still in college, Elisse and I had discussed the name "Ashton" for a son if and when we had children. When I pulled the dollar bill out with the name "Ashton" written across it, I knew right then and there all would be okay, and eventually we would have a normal life with kids and the whole package.

To this day, that dollar remains framed in the room of my first son and will always serve as a reminder of how no matter how uncertain things are, there is always a "greater" plan of which we are unaware.

The "Ashton-dollar" was a great reminder and sign that all would be okay…eventually, but there was still much uncertainty that lie ahead. This was most apparent for me at night time, which had proven to be much harder than day time. Attempting to fall asleep without the comfort of the monitors and the nurses just steps away was very difficult. My "code-blue" experience was very fresh in my mind, and I was fearful of what would be almost certain if I didn't wake up the next morning. There was no "code-blue" service, nor any "nurse-call" buttons in our room – we were all alone, and that was extremely unnerving at the time. Eventually, I began to realize I would wake up in the morning, as I wasn't as sick as I had been in the hospital or I would still be there. Furthermore, I was over mucositis, so there wasn't any reason to worry about airway obstruction. Aside from being nervous about going to sleep and unable to wake up in the morning, it was absolutely wonderful to be home and in my own house and not tied to an IV pole any longer. I could now start focusing on recovery and getting back to a normal life.

Although I wanted nothing more than to get back to normal, it was virtually impossible to do so at this point. Some of my electrolyte levels (magnesium and potassium) were low enough that I needed a six-hour infusion every other day to keep them in range, requiring a return to the outpatient clinic three to four times a week. Thank God, and Lori, who was there and able to accompany me to the hospital and sit and keep me company during those long infusion days. Being tied, yet again, to the hospital, only this time only a few days a week, still made it difficult to return to work and the other aspects of a normal life.

Eventually my electrolytes normalized and about three weeks after being discharged from the hospital, I contacted my work and was scheduled to return to work the following week. Not too bad, I remember thinking, considering at first being told I'd be out for at least six months. Per the policy at work, I had to be able to work two full consecutive 30 hour work weeks before being returned to my full salary level; however, up until that time I would be paid my salary but at the hourly rate for the hours I was able to work. I didn't think this would be an issue, and I returned to work ready to begin my first of two "30-hour" work weeks.

My manager was super cool as was the company, I hadn't even worked for them for three months when I got diagnosed, and all of my medical bills had been paid for thus far. I even received a raise while I was in the hospital. I really wanted to show them my gratitude and wanted to get back to work as soon as possible. My manager told me to take it easy and that I didn't have to push myself to impress anyone and told me to only work when I was able to, saying to leave when I felt I was done. I attempted this for about two weeks, and was only able to work half days before I was both mentally and physically exhausted. My manager brought me in the office and said he appreciated my efforts and realized how important it was for me to get back to normal, but with their policy, I would be able to make more money going back on disability because with disability I was making 60% of my salary which was more than what I was making working at an hourly rate and only being able to work 20 hours per week. Although, this felt like a defeat, I realized he was right and I needed to do what was best for Elisse and me, plus with me being at home, I could regain more strength and come back when I was closer to 100%.

The next few months proved difficult for me. Although it was nice staying home and regaining my strength, there is only so much "Judge Judy," "Maury Povich," "Rikki Lake," and Bob Barker one person can watch, and I was just about tapped out. Elisse was working during the day and Lori had returned home to Virginia. Lori stayed with us for a little over a month to assist until I was stronger and more self-sufficient. The time she was with us provided much solace for me, as I could see how Elisse and Lori were becoming close friends, perhaps even like sisters themselves. This was yet another way this diagnosis actually proved to be a gift, as leukemia and transplant not only brought Lori and me closer together, but also formed a bond between Elisse and her that seemed unbreakable, as both of them were working towards the same goal – my recovery.

Over time, I was beginning to have more good days than bad. My strength significantly improved, as did my appetite. I was now able to mow my lawn in about 30 minutes, and able to eat "double" bacon cheese burgers again. My hospital visits slowed to monthly check-ups and I felt I had definitely made the right choice. My six-month check-up was right around the corner and I was ready to return to work fulltime. This visit was an important one, because at this visit I would be having my chimerism checked.

With transplants, remember the purpose is to irradiate the malignant cells in the bone marrow and replace them with healthy new non-malignant bone marrow from a donor. Chimerism comes from the word Chimera which had a mythological creature that was a mix of several beings, so a "chimerism" test is a blood test looking at what percentage of my blood cells is donor and what percentage is me, and as expected, I was 100% donor. This was great news as, although this was the case at 30 days post-transplant, which is unusual, this confirmed that the graft was holding and I could start coming off my anti-rejection meds and my visits would now taper to three month check-ups. At this visit, I had also requested a "return to work" note from Dr. Rosenfeld, although I had now been back working fulltime for about a week, HR informed me they needed it for their records. I returned to work and handed HR my return-to-work note and went about my day completing my first week back at work.

I now realized how right the transplant coordinator was when she told me it would most likely take about six months for me to return to what would be considered normal, and sure enough, here I was six months later having completed my first week of work since this ordeal began.

The following Monday, week #2, I walked back to my corner office with a view, sat down in my chair, started my computer and began reviewing some training materials. My boss was out on assignment the first half of the day, and in walked our department director, my boss's boss. He asked that I come down to his office for a minute if I had a chance, and as I followed him down to his office, I remember wondering if he was going to talk to me about a promotion. Prior to my diagnosis, my manager had mentioned they were looking to replace my partner and that was the main reason I was hired, aside from me being in a fraternity at Texas Tech, which made them suspect I would be "fun" to work with, and I was fun.

When we got to his office and sat down, he asked me how I was doing and how I was feeling. I told him I was feeling good; my strength had returned; and I was glad to be getting back to work, as I was getting a bit stir crazy staying at home all day. He told me he was glad I was feeling better and back at work and that they had been waiting for my return. He then looked me straight in the eye and told me unfortunately they had to make some cuts and my position was being eliminated effectively immediately. He said there was nothing they could do and he hated to have to give me the news and that my boss wasn't aware this was happening and it would be a shock to him as well. I was escorted back to my office where a box was sitting on my desk. I was instructed to fill it with my personal belongings after which I was then escorted to a conference room where there were about 150 other people who had just heard the same news.

As I sat in the large room with everyone else who had just heard the same news, I remember thinking, "wow – was this really happening?" I had just handed my doctor's note in releasing me back to work a few days ago, had been through chemo, transplant, had just bought a house, and now I was unemployed listening to some jackass, who was still employed, telling all of us how we need to ask for 10% – 20% more while interviewing for my next job and that this event today, will end up being a positive rather than a negative...

I sat through the rest of the "exit interview" and left before noon, still wondering how we were going to make it on Elisse's salary alone, and we wouldn't have had it not been for credit cards, Lori's contributions, and a few miracles.

Unemployment lines would be my next destination, and I would spend most of the next day learning how to find another job; resume strategies; and how to do a job search. These were all requirements to ensure I received the maximum unemployment benefit of approximately $540 per week, a far cry from the near $50K annual salary I was making just moments before.

The hardest thing about being unemployed, with the exception of being broke, was how bored I was with all the time

I had on my hands. This was the beginning of the telecom crash, and I wasn't having any luck in finding a job. With the extra time on my hands, I decided to go back to school. I wanted to make myself more marketable by becoming Cisco Certified and began taking night classes at the local community college.

This pattern of looking for employment by day and taking classes by night became my life, and after about four months of driving to just about every telecom company in DFW to hand them my resume, I finally landed a job with a small telecom company in Carrollton – about 20 miles from home. My new job paid a little more than $9.00 per hour, again, not close to what I was making, but it was a job nonetheless, and I was glad be working again.

Although this job was in the telecom field, it was a far cry from the systems engineering I was doing after college, and similar to what I was doing during college. I was responsible for installing network cable for various clients who hired the company to build their computer networks. I did this for about two months, when the president of the company one morning told my supervisor he needed me to do some work with him that day. I thought this was my chance to prove my worth and attempt to get back to my former salary.

When we arrived at his house and stepped out of the car, I quickly realized just how wrong I was. He directed me to get his mower out of his shed and mow, edge, and hedge his lawn, as he was having a party later that evening. I was absolutely floored at this ass of all asses, but this was 2000, at the heart of the telecom crash, and I needed the job, so I pressed, or rather "mowed" on. After I finished his lawn, as a consultation prize I suppose, he invited me to the party. At the party as he laughed it up while commenting on how nice a job I did on his lawn, I just sat there, said I was classically trained, and continued drinking all of his expensive alcohol.

Needless to say, it wasn't long before I moved on to other employment; although doing pretty much the same thing – network installs. The next place I was employed for about three months; and the next another four months. As a job would get complete, layoffs would occur, and this pattern would keep continuing for a little more than a year.

It was clear to me at this point, I was now suffering from "recurrent layoffitis" and after attending several Cisco classes, I knew I needed to pursue a more advanced, more focused degree utilizing what I had previously learned in my Computer Science classes at Tech coupled with the Cisco classes I was currently taking. I decided to pursue a degree in Electrical Engineering at the community college where I was taking the Cisco classes.

Meanwhile I was still seeing my doctors and was getting stronger and stronger day by day; feeling more normal as well. With the regained sense of normalcy returning along with the strength, I was experiencing an overwhelming compulsion to "give back." I stumbled back onto the Leukemia and Lymphoma Society (LLS). This was the same organization I had received a thank you note from for my donation a few weeks prior, the same day I was admitted to begin chemo when this journey first started.

LLS is a great organization with numerous resources for patients and families of patients with hematologic malignancies – blood cancers, including Leukemia, Lymphoma, and Myeloma as the main three. They are one of few charities that give the majority, well over 70% of the proceeds to the cause for which they were founded. This is truly evidenced by all the research their donations have helped fund and continue to fund. I went to an event put on by LLS introducing "Team N' Training," which was a charitable program where participants would train for either a marathon, or bikeathon and raise funds through donations.

Elisse and I thought this would be a great idea; it would give us a chance to give back, as well as help us get in better shape while training. Remember, when I went into transplant I weighed 230 lbs and now I was at about 185, so I definitely wanted and needed to get back in shape and work out, and this would be a great start in doing so. We signed up and were excited to start working towards our goal of raising $4,000 each to help fund the cost of the trip to the "Rock N' Roll" Marathon in San Diego, while the rest of the proceeds would benefit LLS. We went to our first meeting, met our coach and trainer and began training and prepping for the marathon – little did we know just how short lived this plan would be.

I had completed several Cisco classes by this time, Elisse and I were training for Team N' Training, I was now taking Calculus (EE degree requirement) and I was still picking up network install jobs here and there, but nothing stable, and nothing with benefits. All of the sudden, kind of gradually, but then kind of acutely as well, over the next couple of weeks, Elisse and I started noticing some strange happenings that were going on with me. I was having some difficulty and pain swallowing food (dysphagia), and some intermittent low-grade fevers. I went to my infectious disease doctor, Dr. Howard Kussman, who had now become my primary care physician and internist. As a cancer patient, I had upgraded to specialists and was no longer seeing general practitioners.

Dr. Kussman thought perhaps I wasn't chewing my food enough before trying to swallow and he drew some cultures to check for any infections causing my fevers. He said to keep an eye on the fevers and come back in a week or so to reevaluate. A couple days later, Elisse noticed a white splotchy spot on my arm – very faint, about the size of a half dollar. We didn't really think too much of it. A few more days later, we headed down to my in-laws and the spot had grown and become more noticeable and I was noticing another similar spot on my arm and now my face, although very faint, but still noticeable. I was sitting at the kitchen table at my in-law's house when Elisse looked at me rather matter of factly and said, "You look like you maybe have vitiligo."

When we got back home, I began noticing some white spots on the roof of my mouth and really started to get worried, because if you remember at my initial diagnosis, one of my symptoms was white spots in my mouth. Additionally, I knew if I was going to relapse post-transplant, it would most likely occur within the first two years. Of course, when anyone's concerned about symptoms, the first thing that's always done is the internet is checked, so Elisse consulted with Dr. Google. She searched for post-transplant, white soars in mouth, fever, vitiligo and the most common diagnosis given was "Chronic Graft Versus Host Disease." We printed this information out and brought it with us to my follow-up appointment with Dr. Kussman. Physicians usually are not too pleased when patients attempt to self-diagnose via the internet; however, in this instance Dr. Kussman was in agreement with Dr. Google and quite excited to see his first live case of chronic GVHD. He also admitted he probably wouldn't have even made the diagnosis of chronic GVHD had it not been for Elisse's research and consultation with Dr. Google.

Dr. Kussman then referred me back to Dr. Rosenfeld for evaluation and treatment of my newest condition.

Dr. Rosenfeld confirmed what Dr. Google had suggested indicating I had "de novo" Chronic Graft Versus Host Disease (cGVHD), meaning I had never had Acute Graft Versus Host Disease (aGVHD). My antirejection medication was changed from cyclosporine, which was the standard treatment at the time, to tacrolimus. Tacrolimus, or FK506 as it was called at the time, had been a recently approved novel agent still being investigated in treatment of GVHD then. I was also given a short intensive course of daily high-dose steroids called pulse doses.

Now remember, GVHD is the result of the donor graft (my sister's transplanted bone marrow) attacking the host – ME, and it can attack any organ – skin, liver, gut, eyes – you get the picture, so it was a little frightening and unnerving now that this was happening to me. Although I was concerned, Dr. Rosenfeld did remind me that a little GVHD is good, because of what's called "graft versus leukemia" (GVL) – the result of the graft seeking out and destroying any lingering leukemic cells that were hanging around inside me. Though GVL is a positive side effect, GVHD getting out of control can be very dangerous, so we had to keep it in check by adding the pulse steroids and switching to tacrolimus.

Roughly two weeks went by, my fever had resolved and my throat pain had resolved, as well as the mouth soars; however, now my splotchy skin had become more widespread sporadically covering both arms and legs. Walking also became difficult for me, especially first thing in the morning or after sitting for a long period. I would have to take about 100 or so small steps before I was able to make a normal stride.

These new complications resulted in me returning to see Dr. Rosenfeld, and his first choice was to start me on a therapy using UV light, called photopheresis. Now remember, GVHD is caused by the new transplanted immune system recognizing my whole body as foreign, thus attacking it, and it's the T-cells that are responsible for that role, as they are the cells responsible for recognizing self-vs-non-self, or foreign entities, i.e., ME – and attacking those foreign entities – again ME.

Photopheresis works by running blood through a machine which removes the T-cells and kills them by exposing them to UV light, before the blood is returned to the body. Now this was a relatively new treatment at the time, and Dr. Rosenfeld felt this was my best chance and offered the least amount of side effects, as it wasn't really a systemic therapy and wouldn't completely suppress my immune system. Unfortunately, or rather fortunately come to find out later, my insurance company refused to pay for this novel treatment and said I had to fail another more standard of care cGVHD treatment before they would approve a new one like photopheresis.

Rosenfeld's next choice was to use pentostatin which would significantly suppress my immune system and the T-cells causing the GVHD, so this was added to my GVHD regimen. Now this greatly complicated things because this was a six-hour infusion given twice a week every other week, but it was a necessary evil. My vitiligo was spreading, my ability to walk was becoming more and more compromised, and although I had a very mild case of cGVHD, it could certainly turn to a more serious and even fatal case if it began effecting other organs, and certainly would, if left untreated. After about two weeks of pentostatin, the Vitiligo stabilized and stopped spreading.

Even though the other symptoms of cGVHD had resolved and the vitiligo had stabilized, I was still having difficulty walking and this made it impossible to continue training for the marathon. I couldn't walk normally, and there was no way I was going to be able to make any attempt at running. Unfortunately, Elisse and I would have to pull out of the "Team N' Training" event; although disappointed as we were, we were still able to raise almost $4000 for LLS, and that softened the blow a bit.

Fortunately, although I had to stop with Team N' Training, I was still able to be involved with LLS by joining their "First Connections" program. First Connections matches former patients with newly diagnosed patients in order to mentor, listen, and answer questions they might have. I certainly wished I had known about this when I was first diagnosed, but at least I could provide assistance to someone getting ready to embark on the journey I had been on thus far. It was also becoming apparent to me, studying calculus was difficult while having a six-hour infusion twice a week every other week, so I dropped calculus and said I would return after I completed the pentostatin treatment. My plans for EE degree would have to be put on hold for the time being now.

As my pentostatin treatments continued, eventually my leg pain improved, but my walking was still a bit sluggish, as was my search for meaningful employment. As a few more months went by, it became painfully obvious I was working, rather attempting to work, in a "layoff prone" industry. It was imperative I find another line of work, perhaps start over and find something else to pursue. I had no idea where to start or what to do, as I had been working in Telecom since my Junior year in college, and had no idea what else I could do. I needed something more stable than telecom and had to find something with health benefits. We were fortunate to have health insurance coverage through Elisse's employer, but I couldn't risk being without benefits if something happened with her job. I was still frequenting the doctor's office due to my cGVHD, and I was taking several expensive prescription drugs.

After a few more weeks of working in the faltering telecom industry while intermittently standing in the unemployment line, I was able to land a job with Argenbright Security. You might not recall, but Argenbright Security was the company responsible for just about all of the airport security at the time of the attacks that took place on 9-11. The company came under quite a bit of scrutiny due to security failures that were discovered in light of the attacks, so needless to say, I was a bit concerned about this, especially given the layoff prone industry I was attempting to jump out of. Irrespective of this concern, I couldn't have been happier to have a more permanent job with benefits. To add to my elation, I would be making a little over $11.00 per hour, which was a good deal more than I was making in the telecom industry doing network installs.

My excitement and joy over my new-found security job was short lived. It didn't take long before I began to absolutely hate what I was doing and the associated stigma with being a security guard, a.k.a. "rent-a-cop" with laughable power. Not to knock any security guards out there, it just wasn't for me. I felt demoralized when I put on my uniform and security badge, but that job gave me a benefit I never could have foreseen, something beyond what medicine could do for me at that time.

As a security guard, I had three different posts: 1) cameras – where I would basically monitor the activity across 60+ cameras throughout the complex; 2) guard tower – where I would key people into the complex who were visitors, or who forgot their badge, or needed directions; and 3) patrol – where I'd walk the grounds all shift long, checking offices, and assisting people. Each guard would be given two posts per day and would work each post for four hours. When I was on "patrol," I literally walked non-stop for four hours, with the exception of a 30 minute lunch and a 15 minute break – the rest of the time was all walking. That amount of walking served as a type of physical therapy for me and got my mobility back to 100%.

I worked at that job for about four months before my next dream job came through. I was hired by a large company with great benefits where I could move up through the ranks. I was now working at a very large title company that employed about 3000 people. My new job with First American Title Company came with a $2.00 per hour bump in compensation. I started out in a call center environment but within a year, I was promoted to a job with even better pay and more responsibility. Things were definitely looking up in the employment and career departments now.

A little over 2.5 years had now passed since transplant – my GVHD treatment was stopped about a year prior when, Dr. Rosenfeld left, or was rather forced out of his practice. Apparently, he and the administration butted heads quite a bit and he ended up losing. I didn't find this out until I went in for my 1.5-year check-up, and I was seeing a new doctor from Baylor – Dr. Edward Agura.

It was such a different experience with this new doctor – as he spent 1.5 hours with me wanting to know how everything was going with me and how I was handling everything and if

I had any questions. Dr. Rosenfeld usually spent about 15 minutes with me during an office visit and was in and out and on to the next patient. Compared to Dr. Agura, he did not have much bedside manner, but nonetheless he did save my life and I, to this day have the utmost respect for him.

At that time, I was given the option to continue with Dr. Rosenfeld or switch to the Baylor group and keep seeing Dr. Agura. I asked how many patients were staying with Dr. Rosenfeld, and Dr. Agura mentioned none so far. Dr. Agura's bedside manner impressed me and he seemed genuinely concerned and interested in how I was doing. I also didn't want to tie Dr. Rosenfeld to Medical City Dallas, if I was the only patient he needed to see, so I jumped and decided to continue seeing Dr. Agura.

A couple of weeks went by and I returned to the clinic for my next round of pentostatin, and I saw another Baylor doctor, Dr. Brian Berryman, who became the new Transplant Director at Medical City Dallas. At that visit, Dr. Berryman mentioned he had talked with Dr. Agura, whom I saw two weeks prior, and they both felt it was better for me if I stopped the "systemic" therapy for cGVHD – tacrolimus and pentostatin. The amount of cGVHD I had was very mild and the risk associated with staying on these meds far outweighed the benefits.

These drugs by design were utilized to suppress, or weaken my immune system because it was this "new" immune system that was causing the cGVHD; however, a weakened immune system can increase the risk of infection. I of course agreed if they felt it wasn't worth the risk to continue these meds and they weren't really helping anymore anyway. The only symptom I had was the vitiligo and it had stabilized and stopped spreading.

The decision was clear, so the GVHD meds were stopped. I was concerned a bit about the vitiligo, as I was a little self-conscious about it at the time. People would come up to me asking what happened, or asking if I had gotten badly burned, and it was bothersome always having to explain it. I asked both Dr. Agura and Dr. Berryman what were the chances of my skin returning to normal. I was told it was hard to say for sure, but only time would tell, and Dr. Berryman referred me to a colleague of his, Dr. Jennifer Cather, who was, and still is, a dermatologist experienced with cGVHD.

Simply put, the cause of the vitiligo was cGVHD, but the science behind it was fascinating, as it was my sister's T-cells (now mine), sporadically attacking and killing the melanocytes – cells responsible for making pigment in the skin. This wasn't happening to all the melanocytes, or I would have been suffering from albinism, where all pigment is gone. This is why only certain areas (splotches) lacked any pigment, thus producing this splotchy like pattern. As I was explaining this to Elisse, she asked if I had ever thought of going to medical school and if I really thought I was going to be happy with the EE degree. At the time I kind of brushed her off and didn't really think too much about it. Medicine and especially this field of medicine had become extremely interesting to me, but going back to pursue medical school seemed a pretty daunting task, especially for someone of my "scholarly" past.

A little time had passed and I received my first call regarding a match from LLS's First Connections program requesting me to call Richard, a newly diagnosed patient. LLS asked me to talk with him and share my experience and answer any questions he may have. I first talked with Richard over the phone, and he wanted me to come to his hospital to meet him in person. In his hospital room, he told me one of his friends at work mentioned she had a neighbor from college who had just recently gone through a bone marrow transplant and he should talk to him. Richard said he was planning on it, but wanted to connect through the First Connections program first and contact his friend's friend later. As we continued to talk, Richard mentioned his employer, Interstate Batteries, was a family based company and highly supportive. Upon hearing that Richard worked for Interstate Batteries, I realized his friend was actually our mutual friend, Kelley, who was my neighbor in college, and I was the individual Kelley had recommended he speak with.

After Richard and I finished our visit, he thanked me and said I truly scared the hell out of him, but he nonetheless was happy we had a chance to visit. Elisse also came with me to the hospital to meet with Richard and his wife to share her perspective and speak about being a caregiver. Richard was the first person I talked to and shared my experience with, and I'll never forget the overwhelming feeling of gratitude I experienced in being able to shed some light and remove some of the uncertainty I knew they were facing.

After we got home from visiting Richard and his wife, Elisse again brought up the idea of me pursuing medical school. It was evident to her given how passionate I was about leukemia and how much I had already learned just by being a patient and going through transplant. Elisse couldn't really see me enjoying setting up computer networks in the future, as I certainly don't discuss computer lingo in my spare time and computer programming isn't really a hobby of mine. I asked her if she was being serious and she said she absolutely was. I reminded her what kind of student I was at Tech, on scholastic probation twice, stretching a 4-year degree into 6.5 years, graduating with a 2.1 cumulative GPA – not exactly the stellar student here.

Elisse could see I was having serious reservations and doubts about pursuing medical school, but explained I was a different person now and I was extremely passionate about this field. I had been a patient and had already learned so much. My focus had now changed. I began to think maybe she was right. I had actually always been interested in science and medicine and felt maybe I could do this after all. I began to really ponder this and started to feel maybe this was the reason for my leukemia diagnosis – who better to be your "transplant doctor" than a former transplant patient? The first thing I needed to do though was look into the logistics of this and see just how possible this was for me.

I enjoyed my experience meeting with Richard and felt I could make a difference with a career in medicine. Unfortunately, Richard didn't get his second chance. Richard was the first and only patient whose funeral I attended. He contracted a line infection in his port used for the photopheresis treatment he was undergoing for his GVHD. Photopheresis was the very treatment I was supposed to start for my cGVHD, except my insurance had denied it.

David Copperfield – 3/10/01 – 8 days earlier I was discharged from the hospital.

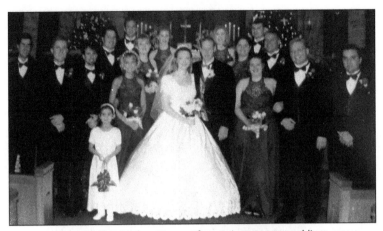

Renewal of vows about 1 year after our impromptu wedding.
This is with our original wedding party.

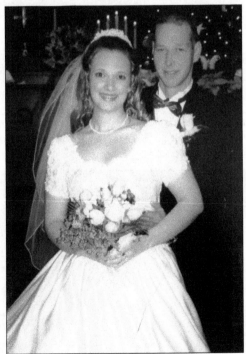

I was about 170 lbs at this point

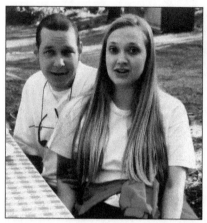

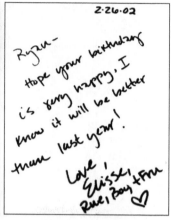

2.26.02

Ryan –
Hope your birthday
is very happy. I
know it will be better
than last year!

Love,
Elisse,
Rae, Boy + Fru ♡

Our delayed honeymoon in Lake Tahoe

You got that right!

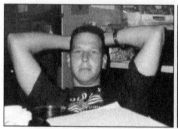

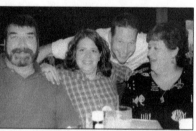

*About a year post-transplant,
pre-GVHD – starting to get
my weight back now*

*Parents, Lori, and I celebrating
1 year post transplant*

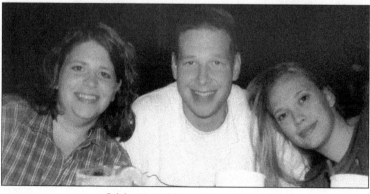

Celebrating with my sister and Elisse

Progress Note

Craig S. Rosenfeld, MD
Texas Cancer Center
at Medical City Dallas
7777 Forest Lane, D-220
Dallas, Texas 75230

Patient:	Woelfel, Ryan	MedRecNum:	
Dictate:	02/17/02	Visitation:	02/15/02
TScribe:	02/21/02. Ajy		

I had a family meeting with Ryan Woelfel and his wife. We talked to the patient and his wife concerning options for therapy for lichenoid chronic graft-versus-host disease. In previous meetings, we discussed the options of Pentostatin, photophoresis, and steroid-based regimens.

Since our last visit, I had spoken to the medical director of Ryan's plan. It was obvious that there was going to be a delay in obtaining approval of the entire therapy of photophoresis. Therefore, I told Ryan we would start him on a regimen of pulse Solu-Medrol and FK-506, as outlined by the Hopkins Group.

I told him we would reassess his response in three months. If he was not responding, we would switch to photophoresis at that time. At the end of the discussion, Ryan and his wife seemed satisfied with the plan. We will see Ryan back Monday to initiate this plan.

Craig S. Rosenfeld, MD

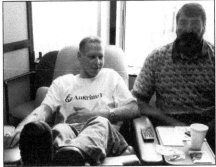

Receiving GVHD treatment

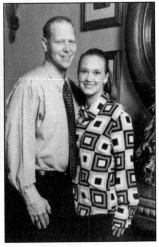

Progress Note

Edward Agura, MD
Texas Cancer Center
at Medical City Dallas
7777 Forest Lane, D-400
Dallas, Texas 75230

Patient:	Woelfel, Ryan	MedRecNum:	469896677
Dictate:	08/09/02	Visitation:	08/09/02
Tscribe:	08/13/02 lkg		

HISTORY OF PRESENT ILLNESS: Mr. Woelfel has a history of acute myelogenous leukemia, currently in remission, status post allogeneic sex mismatched sibling transplant. His recent problems have included cutaneous chronic graft-verses-host disease for which he is being treated with parenteral pentostatin. Patient has received approximately 10 weeks of therapy.

The chronic GVHD is manifested by vitiligo and areas of thickening and scaling in the axillary and inguinal folds. Patient reports no evident improvement of his symptoms since starting pentostatin.

In addition, the patient reports having developed a blurry visual fields. Dr. Rosenfeld had apparently spoken to a neuro-ophthalmologist, Dr. Bingewald at ex. 7684, who had suggested an MRI. This has not yet been arranged. The patient describes his symptoms as blurriness involving the visual fields of the left and right eye.

SOCIAL HISTORY: Patient is returning to work as a computer network specialist. He previously worked in the telecom industry. He is reluctant to give evidence of his prior disease and also to miss work for fear of losing his new job.

PHYSICAL EXAMINATION:

GENERAL: A young healthy male with areas of vitiligo on the arms, chest, face and back.

SKIN: Shows areas of flaking, dryness and loss of elasticity in the folds of the anti-cubital fossa, the axilla, the popliteal fossa and over the anterior-iliac spines.

HEENT: The oral pharynx is benign. The fundoscopic exam is normal.

LABORATORY DATA: CBC shows hematologic remission.

IMPRESSION:
1. Acute myeloid leukemia with remission indices, no evidence of disease recurrence. Chimerism studies have demonstrated full-donor chimerism.
2. No active infectious disease problems, continues on prophylaxis.
3. GVHD, chronic, limited with no obvious response to pentostatin. This drug was therefore stopped and the plan is to observe the patient expectantly. Long-term steroid use is not desirable in this young man, although prednisone is the main stay of therapy for chronic graft-verses-host disease. It could be, however, that a program of mycophenolate and/or sirolimus may provide adequate disease control. If his disease progresses over this next observation period, he will be treated accordingly.
4. Visual field problems. I suspect this may be an ocular neurotoxicity from the pentostatin and may improve. We will call the neuro-ophthalmologist to discuss the MRI procedure.

Edward Agura, MD

CHAPTER 8: NEW FOCUS

Me and medical school ... two words I never thought would be used in the same sentence, but yet here I was, wondering if this would be feasible, not only at my current age of 28, but also given the kind of student I was prior to this journey. Cost as well played a factor in this decision, as I knew medical school would not be cheap and I knew I wouldn't be able to work while in school. I had lots of doubts and questions, and I figured the best person to run this by was my current transplant doctor.

Dr. Berryman seemed fairly young and I had built a great relationship with him. He always seemed to be genuinely interested in how things were going with me outside of my post-transplant experience and I trusted his valued insight. At my next visit, I asked him how old he was when he graduated med school, and how old he was now – 36 was his reply. Then he asked if I was thinking about going to medical school now. I told him he had read my mind and I started to pick his brain on the topic.

I explained I was 28 at the time and knew the first step would require me going back to school to take all the pre-med courses I didn't need for my Telecom degree. I anticipated being in my second year of medical school by my 33rd birthday if all went well concerning my pre-med courses and MCAT scores. Of course, the field of medicine I wanted to practice in was the very field that saved my life – bone marrow transplantation. From start to finish, this would be a 9-year program, meaning I would be close to 40 by the time I had become fully licensed to practice. At age 28, 40 seemed so far off, and I wondered if it was even feasible to begin such a long program at this stage in my life. He squashed any concerns I had about age, indicating he had a friend who had started when he was in his 40's and was now practicing medicine and doing what he loved.

The next hurdle for me was the cost, as I didn't really want to bankrupt Elisse and I on this dream I had, although, I had her full support. He said only the first four years would be unpaid, after that, as a resident, I would make a salary, and I could get loans to assist the first four years if needed. Two hurdles down and one to go – my scholarly past. I mentioned I wasn't exactly the best student, barely squeaking by to graduate. I explained my focus in school wasn't education, but having fun and my GPA and transcript clearly showed this. He said medical schools look at more than just GPA now, they look at the overall potential candidate as a whole, taking into account personal experience, MCAT score, drive, and several other factors. He said if I study hard and do well on the MCAT, I'd be a shoe in, considering what I had just been through.

So, that was that, and now I had a new focus – medical school – and I was determined to get there. First things first. I needed to get in contact with an academic advisor to start working on the framework and get a plan down on paper. The University of Texas at Dallas (UTD) is where this process would first begin. The first thing discussed was the number and type of classes I would need to take to prepare me for medical school. These classes were not just suggestions to merely get me prepared, they were required courses necessary to take in order to apply and be considered for medical school. Although I had already obtained a Bachelor's degree, it was in Telecommunications, and the Bachelor of Arts degree in telecom at Texas Tech didn't require any of the classes medical school requires. All in all, it was looking as if I had an additional 44 hours of course work ahead of me. Daunting this may seem; however, all the coursework was in Biology and Chemistry. This was actually a plus for me because I had always been strong in the sciences, so I wasn't discouraged...yet.

Had I been just a student at this point, this amount of coursework would take about 1.5 years to complete. This was not the case for me, as I was now gainfully employed again with benefits, working about 60-70 hours per week. Additionally, in order to take the upper-level courses, I would have to complete the lower-level ones first, and I would only be able to do so when they were offered. This added great complexity, but little did the advisor know, I had already thought of this and had a solution. I would simplify this by taking only one or two classes per semester. Sure this would take more time to complete, but I didn't want to overload myself and felt this plan was more manageable. Given my tenure at Tech, it was more important to do well now by focusing on a few classes at a time, rather than biting off more than I could handle, which could result in me repeating my educational past. This, of course, I wanted to avoid. I really needed to do exceptionally well this time around and show I was a more focused student and could handle the rigors of med school.

My balloons of excitement and encouragement were quickly deflated as I listened to the advisor explain my plan had several flaws. One of things medical schools consider is the rigor of the applicants' course load compared to their GPA. To demonstrate this, I would need to take a heavy load of courses rather than one or two per semester. She said if I did well in the course work, but only took one or two classes, it would be looked down upon because the course load wasn't rigorous enough. This would lead to serious doubt by the admissions board that I could in fact handle medical school, regardless of how well I did in the classes. I was at a total loss at this point. Here I was a whole one day into this new journey and already being told my only real chance of realizing med school was to essentially quit my job and become a full-time student. This was an impossibility for me. I had no choice but to work. I had a mortgage to pay. Health insurance was a must. In walks much discouragement and uncertainty, but little did I know, something, or someone, would walk in and refocus me sooner than later.

Although med school was still on my mind, it wasn't quite as paramount as it had been prior to my meeting with the UTD advisor. This wasn't because I had given up, I mean yes, I was discouraged, but I was still determined to find a way to get there. The enrollment period had already passed, so I had some more time to figure things out. The timing of this ended up working out, because at this point, I was discussing with Dr. Cather various potential treatment options for my cGVHD induced vitiligo. I was very pleased with her and could tell right away she had a lot of experience in dealing with cGVHD. Like Dr. Berryman, she too seemed genuinely concerned with how I was doing post-transplant, and how I was specifically handling the vitiligo.

I was honest and upfront with her and explained it bothered me a little but at this point, I was looking at it as a reminder of what I had been through more so than anything else. Nonetheless, I was here and through our discussions, there were basically two options of treatment – PUVA or Narrowband. PUVA was more effective. However, the psoralen (the 'P' in PUVA) had been known to potentially cause liver failure. Narrowband on the other hand was basically PUVA, but without the psoralen, so given the issues I had with my liver during transplant, the decision was easy. I opted for Narrowband.

I had my first treatment a little more than a week after Dr. Cather and I discussed it, and it was a little strange to say the least. The treatment consisted of standing in what seemed to be a tanning bed, while being exposed to UVA light at a high intensity. The UVA light generated from the machine would kill the T-cells in my skin that were seeking out and destroying certain melanocytes that were responsible for producing pigment. The experience in the booth was like that of what you would expect from a tanning booth, only obviously way more intense.

The strangest experience with the narrowband treatment was the attire, or lack thereof rather. While in the booth, the only piece of clothing I was afforded was a very large sock. Similar in fashion to the hit SNL song Timberlake and Samberg sang, except instead of "...in a box....," it was "in a sock." This large sock was necessary as it would protect me from getting ultra-burned in a very sensitive area. It was a bit surreal though, I must admit, to be standing in the room with nothing but a sock on when the nurse came in to get me in the booth – a necessary evil I suppose. Initially, this treatment was two times a week with 10 seconds in the booth, but eventually tapered to once a week reaching up to a maximum three minutes in the booth.

The treatment seemed to be going well and I was overall pleased with the results. I was glad Dr. Berryman had put me in contact with Dr. Cather. Not only was she an expert with cGVHD of the skin, she was also an infallible diagnostician.

She had an amazing eye and ability to diagnose based on a mere glance at first, but always followed up by confirmatory biopsy. Not only would this prove beneficial to me now, at this time post-transplant, but also years later as well.

I was about two years post-transplant around this time when I very acutely started feeling what I can only describe as a constant bee sting in the center of my back. I had no idea where it came from, but it came out of nowhere and I was in the shower when I noticed it. I jumped out of the shower, grabbed Elisse and asked her what was there and if she could see anything. She was absolutely no help at all. To her credit though, she was not an infallible skilled dermatologist.

The next thing I grabbed was the phone. Dr. Cather worked me into her busy schedule that day and within a couple hours I was in front of her diagnostic eye. She looked at my back, the very same back Elisse had looked at a couple of hours prior, and said I had shingles. Now for me the shingles wasn't that bad, and I'm not sure if that's because in comparison to transplant, nothing really seemed that bad, or if I just had a mild case. Either way, she put me on an antiviral and within two weeks, it was over with no lingering evidence I ever had it.

With shingles behind me now and the Narrowband treatment going well, the thought of medical school again rose to the forefront of my brain. It was at a routine check-up with Dr. Berryman, a little over two years post-transplant, when through our discussions, my efforts to pursue medical school had been restored. The first question he asked was how the med school tract was going. I told him how my first meeting went and he shook his head saying what I had heard was ridiculous and not to be discouraged. He said when he was in medical school, he sat on the admission's interview board, and the information I had been given was from an undergraduate advisor. Dr. Berryman said it would be better to go right to the source and gave me the contact information of the Director of Admissions at UT Southwestern Medical School – Dr. Scott Wright. He told me to contact him requesting a sit-down meeting to share my story with and to ask for any advice he may have regarding pursuing med school. It took all of a week for me to get this meeting set and with transcripts in hand, my story on my tongue, and passion in my heart, I slowly began unfolding my recent life story.

Dr. Wright sat there very attentive as I told my story. He looked over my transcripts. He said he could definitely see my passion and felt inspired. We discussed the hurdles I would have to overcome and he agreed I had received some bad and outdated information regarding pursuing med school. Like Dr. Berryman had said, he confirmed they look at more than just the GPA/MCAT score and consider the applicant as a whole. He said, and even advised, taking some of the pre-med courses at a community college in order to defray some of the cost I was sure to incur as I embarked on this task. He also mentioned that taking a heavy load to demonstrate I could handle to rigors of med school wasn't necessary and probably was counter-productive in my case, given this was already demonstrated in that I was currently working 70+ hours/week.

All of this information was in complete contradiction to what the undergraduate advisor at UTD had mentioned, and I was glad I had gone straight to the source. Our initial 30-minute meeting lasted a little over two hours and the advice I had been given was invaluable. I again was indebted to Dr. Berryman for putting me in contact with him. As our meeting came to an end, he thanked me for sharing my story and my interest in pursuing med school. He then made me promise I would get back in contact with him after I had completed my pre-med courses, prior to applying. Given the number of applicants, he wanted to be sure to pull my application when it crossed his desk. I was overjoyed and filled with encouragement and determination as I left his office, and was excited to get started.

After speaking with Dr. Wright, I knew I had some flexibility regarding where I took my classes and could take them where my schedule allowed. The first class available for me to take was General Chemistry 1. It was offered at UT Arlington and it was even offered during the summer in an accelerated format. I was a little apprehensive about taking the class in an accelerated format over the summer, but I felt it couldn't be that bad, as it was Gen Chem, and I always enjoyed the sciences.

After the first couple weeks, it was becoming quite apparent the only acceleration that was occurring in this accelerated class, was me getting the hell out. Perhaps jumping into an "accelerated" summer Gen Chem class roughly 11 years since I had had any chemistry, in high school mind you, wasn't the smartest option. This was especially true when you combine the amount of work I was doing outside of school. I took Honor's Chemistry in high school, but I was now learning about electron configuration and how electrons would jump into different orbitals depending on how energized they would become through various bonding and reactions. I was solving problems in molarity and molality, and balancing heat reactions. This might as well have been a foreign language I was learning, and in a way, it was I suppose. If I had been taught this prior, I remembered none of it. It wasn't just the material being new to me that made the class unworkable, but the very structure of the class as well. Being the class was accelerated, the lecture was two hours daily, five days per week and the lab was four hours, one day per week. I was living in Plano, working in Dallas and going to class in Arlington, so basically, I would drive about an hour in the morning to work, then drive 30 minutes to class after work and then drive an hour back home after class, and I was doing this five days a week. Note, none of this included any study time, which I was using my weekends for. This wasn't working out too well and my grades in the class were starting to suffer. The adviser's words were screaming at me regarding GPA, GPA, GPA. I had no choice but to drop the class and take a "W" in order to save my GPA, and take it again when it was offered in a normal non-summer, non-accelerated semester.

It was time to see Dr. Berryman again for another check-up. Clinically speaking, I was doing well, so similar to my last check-up, we discussed things outside of my health – pursuing med school and work mostly. I told him as far as pursuing med school, the first class didn't go at all how I had expected, and I ended up having to drop it. He said these classes can be difficult to do well in, especially while working. He stressed taking them in an accelerated fashion, although would save time, would eventually hurt me if I didn't do well in them. I explained I already came to this conclusion and wouldn't be bogging myself down any further.

As for work though, I explained I was ecstatic to be working full-time again and with benefits as well, but my passion wasn't in escrow account balancing. He agreed. I had asked if he knew, or had any suggestions as to how I could break into the medical field – more specifically transplant. I really wanted to work in the very field that saved my life. I had been on the patient side of things and now I wanted to experience what was on the other side of it – the non-patient side. He told me he would ask around at Baylor and see what was out there, if anything, and would let me know. Out of nowhere, he then pulls out his phone and called one of his colleagues – Dr. Joseph Fay.

At the time, unbeknownst to me, Dr. Fay was a god in the world of immunology and bone marrow transplantation. A true pioneer. He brought bone marrow transplantation out from the world of obscurity and into the epicenter of North Texas. He designed, built, and started the Blood and Marrow Transplantation Program at Baylor University Medical Center in Dallas 30 years prior, helping it to become the leading center for blood and marrow transplantation in all of North Texas at present day.

When I had asked Dr. Berryman if he had any suggestions on how I could get my foot in the door in the medical field, I certainly didn't expect him to get on his phone right then and there, but I was sure glad he did. Unfortunately, Dr. Fay didn't have anything at the time as he was really looking for someone with some research experience. I thanked Dr. Berryman and told him he didn't have to call anyone right then and there, but I really appreciated it nonetheless. Then before he "flipped" his phone closed (yes this was the era of "flip" phones), he shocked me again. He called the research manager at Baylor, and then before I knew it, he called the doctor who set up the Blood and Marrow Transplantation Program at UT Southwestern, also in Dallas. He wasn't able to reach them at this time, but left messages with both. He gave me their contact information and said if I didn't hear something back from either of them within the week, to give him a call and he would follow-up. Wow! I cannot express how indebted to him I was. Dr. Berryman didn't have to do any of this. He could have just brushed me off and pretended to be interested in my future plans, but I soon discovered, this was old hat to him. This was just the kind of person he was. Definitely so much more than a doctor and far surpassed any expectations I already had at that point.

It was about one week later, a very long week, when I heard back from both the research manager at Baylor and the transplant group at UT Southwestern. Dr. Robert Collins, the Director of the Blood and Marrow Transplant Program at UT Southwestern wanted to sit down with me and discuss what my plans were for the future. He wanted to get an idea if they had any positions I would fit into in his program. His administrative assistant said she would be calling me within the next month or so to set up an interview. Baylor, on the other hand, wasn't looking too promising as the research manager informed me she only had positions opened for nurses presently. She did say another manager in another research department had an opening and put me in contact with her.

A couple of weeks later, lo and behold, I now had two interviews – one at UT Southwestern and one at Baylor. I wasn't nervous at all, because I was extremely confident. I had just beaten cancer and I was on top of the world again – this was all part of my destiny now. I knew I could provide a unique perspective to patients in this filed, which no other applicant could provide. My interview with Baylor was first and the one with UT Southwestern was set for two days later. At the Baylor interview, I quickly learned I was being interviewed for both the Blood and Marrow Transplant Program and the Solid Organ Transplant

Program. I was honest and upfront with both managers. I told them this was a way for me to break into the medical field and that eventually I was planning on going to medical school with the aspirations of one day becoming a transplant doctor myself. I explained what I had been through and that my passion laid with BMT. However, I would be willing to work in solid organ transplant to get my foot in the door. Again, I stressed I really wanted to be in BMT. I think I mentioned that to them in those exact words at least three or four times, so I'm pretty sure they understood I really, really, really, really wanted to work in BMT.

As the interview was coming to a close, I felt it went really well and I had asked if there were any other applicants or interest in the positions. They informed me they had over 50 applicants and I was the 10th interview with three more to go. I thanked them for their time and again stressed I would really very much enjoy breaking into this field and although I would work for either program, I was hoping for the BMT one. I think they fully got this. I walked out, said thanks again, and headed home, knowing I would be interviewing with UT Southwestern in a couple days.

Those two days came and went and before I knew it, there I was in Dr. Collins's office waiting to see what and if they had any positions available for me. We talked about my diagnosis and treatment. We talked about his interest and where he felt his program was headed. We even talked a little about Baylor and how he knew the program well. Turns out he coincidentally worked at Baylor before leaving to start the program at UT Southwestern, and knew the program well. He also knew Dr. Berryman well, as he happened to be one of the transplant doctors who trained him. He then said something to me that has always stuck with me. He said I was the poster child for BMT and remarked how lucky I was to be sitting in his office having made it through all I had been through. He applauded my efforts at "wanting to give back" and mentioned there at UT Southwestern, although he's a transplant physician, he's really trying to get away from, or at the very least, more fine tune BMT. Dr. Collins mentioned he felt, at the present time, BMT was more of a sledge hammer treatment and he was looking for more of a mallet and chisel. He said they (BMT physicians) must do a better job at transplant because too many people don't make it through. He said it was refreshing for him to have met someone doing so well post-transplant.

Being post-transplant, I've heard this so many times. The transplant doctors, and nurses as well, never see the ones that are doing well post-transplant, they only see the ones doing poorly. We continued to discuss my plans and aspirations and he told me he was glad I had spoken with the folks at Baylor because right then, he didn't have any openings. He said to keep in touch with him, wished me all the luck with med school, and told me if the Baylor opportunity didn't pan out to personally contact him and he would find something for me at UT Southwestern without a doubt. I took what he said to heart, thanked him for his time and headed home.

Now the waiting game had started, and wait I did, but not too long, as about a week – a very long week – I got the call from Baylor. They were offering me the position as a Research Associate in their Blood and Marrow Transplant Program. I was on top of the moon with excitement. I called Dr. Collins at UT Southwestern to let him know Baylor had in fact come through, and thanked him again for speaking with me about potential opportunities at UT Southwestern. He congratulated me, said it was a good program, and told me to contact him if I ever needed anything in the future.

Everything was now starting to come together again. I was overjoyed at getting the opportunity to work in this exciting field I had now become a product of, and with summer ending soon, I was ready to begin taking pre-med courses again. This time around, I was going to attempt to take Biology 1. However, I was going to be taking it in a normal non-accelerated semester. Collin County Community College is where it was offered at the available times that would work with my current work schedule. Remember, I was working 60 to 70 hours per week, so I had to take classes that would fit when and where they were available.

I was way more excited about Biology than Chemistry, as I was always extremely interested in Biology and given what I had just been through, I was even more eager to learn as much as I could about it. I registered for class, and couldn't wait for it to begin, and before I knew it, it had.

I walked into the building straight to the information desk to ask where the class was. They responded by directing me to the class and asking if I needed anything else for the class. I thought to myself, "wow, that was nice to ask if I needed anything else for the class." Then before I could respond, I was asked if I was new to the district and if I had any questions about my students or when my office hours were. I smiled and said, "Nope I was just a student," which was followed with some awkward silence. This was the first time I had been confused as being the professor rather than the student, but it certainly wasn't the last. I attributed it to the distinguished looked my new glasses (side effect of cGVHD) afforded me. In any case, the first day came and went, followed by the first week, then months and before I even knew it, I had now completed my first pre-med course, receiving an "A" no doubt. Definitely a far cry from what my undergrad experience was like at Tech, but now my focus was different.

With the first semester behind me and now three months into my new position as a Research Associate, things were looking up. I was learning so much in my new position. Literally for the first time in my life, work didn't feel like work at all. It was an absolute joy going to work every day in a field I was truly intrigued with and passionate about. I had no idea what all went into transplantation on the back end – the non-patient side.

Every Monday, the program team would all meet and discuss each patient, first those in the hospital, either going through transplant or getting ready to go through transplant. Then we would discuss patients who were waiting to get transplants either because of insurance issues or delays, or those waiting to find matched donors, either siblings or through the National Marrow Donor Program (NMDP). Wednesdays there would be a lunch lecture where HemMalig (hematologic malignancies) and BMT physicians would present cases for discussion. In these meetings, lectures on all aspects of each disease we as a program worked on were given.

Now I had acute myelogenous leukemia (AML), of which there were eight types at the time (now acute leukemia is even more divided into subgroups), but that was just one of the diseases we worked with. In my position, I was fortunate to work and learn about all the hematologic malignancies (blood cancers) – acute leukemia, chronic leukemia, myelodysplastic syndrome, myeloma, hodgkin's lymphoma, non-hodgkin's lymphoma and all the subtypes of each disease. I wasn't only learning about the diseases in and of themselves. I was also learning the pathophysiology of these diseases, the natural history of these diseases, and the natural progression of these diseases. I was definitely a sponge and was absorbing so much information. It was truly an amazing wealth of information I was learning and I felt this would surely prove to be beneficial when in medical school.

The specific team I was on, consisted of a manager (a bio-statistician) and three other research associates like myself – two were foreign doctors, yet we were all equal in our job duties. I felt very fortunate to be working hand in hand with doctors. Although they were foreign doctors, they still proved vital in my training and I was greatly appreciative as they took me under their wings to teach me everything they could regarding these diseases and the treatment thereof.

Our primary focus was to submit data forms to the International Blood and Marrow Transplantation Registry (IBMTR). This was the lifeblood of the Transplant Program, as without the forms being submitted both timely and accurately, the program would not be accredited. Without accreditation, insurance companies wouldn't approve transplants at our center and patients would have to go elsewhere to be treated. These forms consisted of thousands of data points for each patient, at each specific time-point from pre-transplant, through various time-points post-transplant through long-term follow-up, up to and including death.

Each of us was given an equally divided portion of the alphabet (alpha-split) to work on. Each patient that would come in to the transplant program, would be paired up with the member on our team who had the letter of the patient's last name within their respective alpha-split. That team member was responsible for all the data submission for that patient throughout transplant until the patient became lost to follow-up or expired (died).

I was responsible for all data submissions for patients whose last name began with the letters, H – L, S and N. The information that was gathered from our site (Baylor), was entered into the national database. This data, once combined with data gathered from transplant centers the world over, was analyzed to tease out multiple data points, so conclusions could be drawn, ultimately providing better outcomes for patients with these hematologic malignancies. The data would help answer some important questions and quite possibly lead to practice changing ideals. Questions like – Which diseases respond better to which treatment and which different combinations are more effective in certain diseases, while ineffective in others? Does age play an impact – for the patient or the donor, or neither, or both? Does the graft matter – peripheral blood vs. bone marrow? Do certain treatment combinations confer more GVHD, or less? How is overall survival affected compared with a treatment that prolongs disease free survival? If one treatment produces a longer disease free survival, but patients ultimately die as a result of toxicity to the regimen, albeit in remission, does that truly mean that specific treatment is better than the others? Does gender mismatch confer worse outcomes for transplant patients? At what dose of radiation can treatment be effective, without causing worse GVHD, or other long-term effects, such as other malignancies, or pulmonary fibrosis, or congestive heart failure, or diabetes? These were types of questions we were helping to answer. We were literally helping to change practice and how patients were treated. The very regimen used to cure me in fact, isn't even used today by most centers, because of the toxicity associated with it. Remember, I was told the regimen that was being used on me would have killed someone in their 50's. This is a real-time true testament to how this data, once analyzed, could be used, and was used, to change practice to produce better patient outcomes. This, in and of itself, gave me more fulfillment than I ever could have imagined I would ever be able to obtain from a job. I was truly fortunate and I knew this.

In addition to extracting data and entering it as described above, often times and when time would prove available, we would work on ancillary research projects the BMT physicians would assign us to. Within my first month I got my first assignment. I was asked to provide the number of CD34+, CD3+, CD4+, and CD8+ cells in the donated graft to the recipient. Now at the time, I didn't know what any of this meant, what these cells were, and what exactly I was being asked to do. It wasn't long though before I understood exactly what they were and what I was being asked to do and for what purpose. CD34, or "cluster of differentiation" 34, is a protein that's expressed on certain cells (CD34+) and not expressed on others (CD34-), and in this instance, hematopoietic stem cells from the donor that were infused into the patient expresses CD34, meaning they are CD34+. CD3+ refers to cells that activate T-cells, CD8+ refers to cytotoxic T-cells that kill, and CD4+ refers to helper T-cells that send signals (cytokines) to cytotoxic T-cells to bring them to the invading substance, infection, microbe – you get the idea – in order to destroy them. Very, very, very basic immunology here, but basically, I was being asked to find out the number of stem cells, and various types of t-cells that were delivered in the graft the patient received from the donor. This information was important because often times if the number of stem cells

(CD34+) was too low, the patient was at a risk of rejecting the graft because there weren't enough of the donor's stem cells available to effectively engraft, resulting in graft failure. On the other side of it were the T-cells – if there were too many, then the risk of GVHD would rise, but if too few, then the risk of relapse or rejection may rise. This particular study was a retrospective analysis at this point, as the patients had already been transplanted, but the information gathered, could prove or disprove how important or unimportant knowing this information ahead of time would be in producing better outcomes for our patients.

I had a few more months under my belt at work and I was embarking on my second class – General Chemistry 1. It was offered at the community college where I had just completed my Biology 1 class the semester prior, so I was pleased with that. Things were going much better this time around. Could it be the fact it was at a community college? Perhaps. Or could it be it too was a normal semester and not an accelerated one? Who knows. It didn't really matter to me because I was doing great in it and that's all that matters. Second class down and it was a "B" this time, still doing much better than when I was at Tech, and I was working fulltime now as well. I felt good about this and was ready for the next class.

I was nearing my six-month mark now in my new position, and have done exceptionally well in my first two pre-med courses. I had learned so much and was continuing to do so. I still loved what I was doing, but the extra side projects I was assigned to is what really felt like research to me. My next assignment came and it was a little less "clinical," but still important, especially in my long-term goals of getting to med school. There is an annual meeting held at different locations throughout the nation where transplant physicians and ancillary staff from across the globe come to present novel treatments and research they have been working on. The analyzed data from novel treatments under study at various sites are often presented and reviewed against the control, or standard of care treatment and the corresponding outcomes. This "control" is what I, along with the other members on my team, help provide in consort with similar teams like ours at other sites across the globe.

This particular meeting at this point was unique this time compared to prior meetings. Our manager had developed an internal database that mirrored that of the IBMTR's database, but rather than it being international, it was site centered – Baylor specific. This database she developed was extremely beneficial to our BMT docs, and it provided trends they could see within our center allowing them to adjust practices accordingly if need be. My specific task this time was to co-author the abstract our center would be submitting to this international meeting in the coming months. If selected, I would be presenting the poster that would accompany it at the meeting, addressing any questions regarding its use and effectiveness at our center. As I said earlier, although this wasn't really a clinical application, it was still important in my goal of getting into med school, because if it was selected, which it was, then it would be published in a medical journal, which it was, and then, I could list it on my CV/resume as a "publication" I had, which I did.

A few more months went by and, few more, and before I knew it, I was nearing two years at Baylor. All the information I had learned was paying off and the passion I had for working in this field was paying off as well, as I was now the lead in our group. I was now training new members to the group and assisting our manager with some of her duties. This added responsibility was proving to make studying and focusing on school a little difficult, but I was still determined as I was sure med school was in my future. Although work was affecting my studies a bit, I was still managing to do pretty well I thought, and a hell of a lot better than I did at Tech.

I had now completed Biology 1 (A), Gen Chem 1 (B), Gen Chem 2 (B), Physics 1 (C), Physics 2 (C), Organic Chem 1 (C), and now gearing up for Organic Chem 2. Of all these classes, without a doubt, the hardest class, hands down, was Organic Chem 1. To add to this difficulty, I had already begun prepping for the MCAT (Medical College Admissions Test) while I was taking Organic Chem 1, and now I was gearing up to take it within the next few weeks. I had enough of the pre-med courses under my belt to sit for the MCAT and in order to prep, I took one of the preparatory classes. I had been reading all the books and taking the practice test. I felt confident and was ready to take the test – the test that would do nothing at all, but decide the rest of my future.

The test itself was grueling – it was comprised of four sections 1) Physical Sciences, 2) Verbal Reasoning, 3) Biological Sciences, and 4) Writing. Each section was timed and the test altogether took six hours to take. I was completely drained by the end of the test and highly concerned for my score. Of the four individually timed sections, I was able to complete none of them before the time ran out. Given my "less than par" GPA from Tech, combined with my recent grades, from the pre-med courses I had completed, I needed to get at least a 32 (45 is a perfect score), to be somewhat competitive. It was highly doubtful I had achieved that high of a score, or anywhere close to it. In six weeks – six long weeks – that fear became a reality.

Doubling my score would certainly have put me in a better spot, but at a score of 19, I was a far cry from where I needed to be. Nevertheless, I persisted. I felt although my chances were slim to none, I would go ahead and apply. I just needed one interview, just one, and I knew I would be able to get in. I just needed to get face to face with the admissions board, and share my personal experience and passion. I was hoping against hope, but determination and will are powerful driving forces. Med schools look at the whole package remember, not just GPA and MCAT score. Given my score and GPA, my best chance at getting an interview was to try the shot gun approach with my application. I would be applying to as many schools as possible, at the mere hope of one biting. I needed to cast a wide net, and so the grueling process begun.

When applying to med school, you must use a centralized application service, one for Texas – TMDSAS (Texas Medical and Dental Schools Application Service), and one for the rest of the U.S. – AMCAS (American Medical College Application Service). Then each individual school has their own application with questions specific to their school. I was applying to all the med schools in Texas and several out of state – 24 schools in all. So, that's 24 individual applications, each with their own individual specific questions. How I felt I could fit in their specific medical school. Why I wanted to go to medical school. How I felt I fit in with each schools' mission and philosophy. These were in addition to the questions on the centralized applications through TMDSAS and AMCAS. In addition to answering these questions, I had to explain if and why I was, if I ever was, considered "not in good standing" with any institution of higher education. Not in good standing translates to scholastic expulsion or scholastic probation. Of the two flavors, I was of the latter. Probation is much better than expulsion, but in my case, I had to explain why I was placed on probation not once, but twice. First one was easy to explain – I was a freshman from a small town and was experiencing freedom and coming into adulthood via trial and error. The second occurrence came in my "second" junior year. This point in my college tenure was the best personally for me, but the worst for my grades. The first part of the semester, the two friends in the opening story (Chris and Dave) and I pretty much spent our time, all our time, grilling, drinking beer, and attending an occasional class by day, and drinking beer and going out by night. This was pretty much how our semester went for the most part, and it was evident in all of our GPA's, as ours' added together still fell short of a 4.0 – my contribution to the equation was a 0.8. Could I have possibly improved on this GPA? Perhaps, but towards the end of the semester stood before me my biggest obstacle yet to focusing on school – Elisse. Elisse. Elisse. Focus on school – subverted. Clearly explaining "...I spent an entire semester my second junior year getting smashed and meeting a girl...," wouldn't fly, and finding a way to spin this proved difficult.

Equally difficult was collecting all the transcripts I needed to submit, as there were numerous. To capture all the course work I had completed from my initial undergraduate course work up to and including the pre-med course work, my education had spanned across 12 years ('94 – '06) and five colleges at this point – Texas Tech University, the University of Texas at Arlington, Collin County Community College, Southern Methodist University, and the University of Texas at Dallas.

Each University had its own process and associated fee for requesting transcripts. The fees for the transcripts ran around $10 to $30, depending on the school. This cost was nominal; however, keep in mind it was per school, and this certainly wasn't the only cost associated with applying to med school.

I wasn't ignorant to the fact med school would be expensive, but it was eye opening, to say the least, when it came to the expense associated with just getting to that point. I already discussed the transcript request fees I had to pay, but in addition to those, each med school I was applying to required an application fee. This fee ranged anywhere from $25 to $200, again depending on the school. Keep in mind I was applying to 24 schools, so that got pretty expensive pretty fast. These application fees due to each school, were in addition to the application fees associated with each centralized application service – TMDSAS and AMCAS – another $200 each. Keeping with this $200 theme, to sit for the MCAT cost $200. The MCAT prep course I took, another $200? Nope – this class broke that trend as it was $1500. All in all, just the process of applying to med school, prepping for the MCAT, and taking the MCAT totaled just under $5,000. Notice this doesn't take into account the cost of the pre-med courses I had taken up to this point.

Now that I had completed all the applications and transcript submitting and the graduate record explaining and the how I fit with your med school philosophy explaining, I had one final thing to do – contact Dr. Wright, the Director of Admissions at UT Southwestern Medical School, which he made me promise I would do four years earlier when I started this journey. I wasn't sure if he would even remember me, but after I reached his office, I realized it didn't really matter anyway, as he was no longer working at UT Southwestern – he had left a few months prior. So, that was that and all I could do at this point was wait, and wait, and wait, and wait, and wait some more, and then wait a little more. This I did while also working and continuing with classes, as one thing I learned from my advisors was med schools don't like to see any gaps in education.

Organic Chem 2 was the next class I had to take during this time, and believe it or not I was looking forward to it. I had heard horrible things about it and I had known people at Tech who had to change majors or drop out of the University because of the difficulties associated with Organic Chem 2. I wanted to get this class over and done with. Something I learned, almost immediately, in Organic Chem 2 that I still remember to this day – Organic Chem 1 was a cake walk. I never thought this to be true until after my first class in Organic Chem 2. I quickly realized the stories were true and when I somehow, by the grace of God, received a "C," I took it and ran and never looked back.

As I continued with the waiting game for responses from the 24 med schools I had applied to, I had plenty of distractions to keep me occupied. Work at this point was going strong; however, it was starting to bog me down a bit. It was still interesting, but I wanted to do more hands-on research, and less forms. The forms were important and served a purpose in research, but I wanted to work more on ancillary projects and clinical trials or the design thereof. Even more so distracting than my work, was another exam that needed much preparation that was quickly approaching, but not for me. This exam was for Elisse, but it equally distracted me from the med school response waiting game.

Law School was something Elisse mentioned she was interested in while we were at Tech. Soon after graduating, our plans were quickly turned upside down when I was diagnosed and she put pursuing law school on hold. Once I had come out of transplant, and made it out of the woods so to speak, she fervently pursued law school, and now it was time for the BAR Exam. I was extremely proud of her. Not only did she do it while working fulltime, she also commuted two hours daily to complete this task in 3.5 years. Her accomplishment not only benefited both of us financially, but it also gave her a great sense of fulfillment. Her determination, focus, and stick-to-itiveness, not only impressed me, but empowered me to continue on in my pursuit of med school. The timing of this couldn't have been more aptly planned, as while she was in law school, I was completing my pre-med courses. This provided each of us time to study our respective courses without having to worry about the other feeling ignored. We had no time to feel ignored. During the week, we would work and on the weekends we would study – each of us our own subjects.

As Elisse was prepping for the BAR, the class I was taking at the time was by far my most exciting, interesting class to date – Molecular Biology of Cancer. I learned so much in this class, and it really hit home given what I had been through. We delved into the numerous pathways – hundreds upon hundreds – with which cancer uses to thrive and survive. We discussed the body's natural defense to cancer, tumor suppression genes, and ways cancer bypasses those genes, and evades the natural surveillance mechanisms of the immune system. We discussed pathways that were up-regulated, as well as those that were down-regulated, and how when one pathway is targeted by a treatment, how another pathway forms – resulting in the next target for treatment – targeted therapy. It was a highly intriguing class and I was learning so much. It was definitely the impetus to my interest in immunology – the next class I was planning to tackle and looking forward to.

Aside from being a cancer survivor, one of the reasons I was excited about, and did well in, the Molecular Biology of Cancer course, was it somewhat tied into what I dealt with on a daily basis working in cancer research. The bad part about the class though in how it related to work, was it was slowly making me become more and more dissatisfied with my specific role in the research department. Don't get me wrong, I still felt very fulfilled, I just wanted to better "give back" to the field I was working in – the field that had saved my life. I knew the data we were extracting and entering into the international data base, was helping to change practices. Remember, I understood first-hand how important that was, as I stated before concerning the regimen used in my transplant.

This was basic research we were doing, contributing here, as we were providing the "control" – the standard of care – data for all the research studies worldwide in this field. I still enjoyed Baylor and the people I worked with, but I felt at this point, with what I had learned thus far at work and through the pre-med courses I had taken, I wanted more. I soon learned, as I pushed and inquired about my desire of wanting to, not only contribute more, but also learn more, there was a bigger underlying issue at play here. Much like an indolent cancer slowly invades, takes over, and wreaks havoc, this underlying issue I discovered was also behaving in this manner. Unfortunately, ultimately over time, this nasty cancer-like growth that starts small and un-noticeable at first, grows and becomes large and uncontrollable. It effects all sorts of industries and institutions, and can even be deadly to a program if left unchecked. What is this cancer you might ask? I'm quite sure you have faced it as well – the "business side" of things; administration; policies. Now, I know and fully understand there is a business side to everything, as it's money that makes the world go round. Ultimately if something doesn't result in a profit, or at the very least – breakeven, then it can't be sustained. To have a successful business, businesses must have policies and administrations to run those policies. Problems begin to arise though when those policies, although, written in black and white, don't provide for any of the gray that's surely to come up. This was the situation in my case.

I wanted to do more research-based applications other than data extraction and analysis. I wanted to get more into the research of novel treatments, both developing them and studying them. I undoubtedly hit a wall laden with administrative policies. At Baylor, unfortunately at this time, policy dictated I had to be a nurse in order to do the kind of research I was interested in doing. Furthermore, the current structure of the department I was in wouldn't allow any movement in this regard. Although there was a research department and I was doing research, the two were a little separate. I was working with data elements extraction whereas the other was working more with new study drugs and patients – the main difference, one required an RN, one did not. This put me in a tricky spot.

My ultimate goal was med school, so my ultimate fulfillment would come from that; however, if I could break into the type of research involving protocol design and management, I would certainly be in a better position for med school. It was a difficult decision, but I felt I had no choice. I felt the only way to be more fulfilled and be in a better position for med school, was to jump ship at Baylor and look for other opportunities. Coincidentally, around this same time, a former clinic manger in BMT HemMalig at Baylor, now working at UT Southwestern, had recently given my name to their Director of Clinical Research and they contacted me to see if I would be interested in coming aboard at UT Southwestern. Even more so coincidental was at this same exact time, a former nurse in the BMT HemMalig clinic at Baylor, who was now working at US Oncology, had contacted me to see if I'd be interested in working with them.

Just three years ago, I was a patient in this field and now I had two institutions coming to me, inquiring about my interest in joining their organization. I was dumbfounded. I interviewed with both institutions, and the timing of how this all went down definitely worked towards my advantage. The first interview was with US Oncology, and it was for a Regulatory Specialist position. In this position, I would be responsible for submitting new study protocols to a central Institutional Review Board (IRB). This IRB board consists of a group of people, some from legal, some medical, some from outside community, all brought together to review the scientific validity, contribution, feasibility, and the safety of each study submitted. In this position, I would also be writing the consent forms and assist with prepping for internal and external audits of study patient charts. I was excited about this potential. Not only did this feel more like the patient directed research I was looking for, but it was also a 30% pay increase over what I was currently making at Baylor. More pay – icing on the cake. A couple of days went by, an offer from US Oncology came, and I quickly accepted. Now the hard part – telling Baylor.

I felt like I was betraying Baylor, and especially Dr. Berryman. With no practical experience, Baylor gave me a chance, and that certainly wouldn't have occurred had Dr. Berryman not vouched for me. Plus, I really enjoyed working with the people I had been working with over the past three years. My manager was completely shocked, dismayed, and disappointed when I handed in my letter of resignation and 2 weeks' notice. I assured her it had nothing to do with her, but felt, due to the administrative policies currently in place, I had no choice but to jump. My position and learning had become stagnant at this point and I needed a change. I needed to be able to contribute more and delve more into the world of research. I thanked her for giving me the opportunity and then went back to my office.

As I sat down to begin typing the email to alert the rest of the team and physicians concerning my departure, my phone rang. Literally 10 minutes had passed since I handed in my letter of resignation, and the research manager at Baylor was on the phone. This was the same research manager I had talked to when I first came to Baylor, who had no openings in her department for a non-nurse with zero experience. This was the team I was wanting to work on, but because I wasn't a nurse, this wasn't possible given the current policy. This policy was the reason I was leaving and had accepted the position at US Oncology. Little did I know at the time, this was about to change. The Research Manager, who officed right down the hall from me, said she just heard I had resigned. She said she would hate to see me go and asked if she was able to get me a position on her team as a Clinical Research Coordinator, would I reconsider and stay. I told her absolutely, but wasn't sure how that would happen since I wasn't a nurse. She said she needed to make some phone calls and talk to a few people and see if something could be worked out. I explained how appreciative I was, but I had already accepted an offer with US Oncology and didn't want to burn a bridge with them at this point. Additionally, they had offered me 30% over what I was making in my current salary, and I was extremely doubtful Baylor would meet that offer. She said she would have to contact Human Resources to see what they could do in that regard, as the norm is a 10% match, but asked that I give her a week to see what she could work out. A few days went by and she said they were in the process of creating a "non-nurse" Clinical Research Coordinator position, and it was looking promising this was going to happen. The main issue at this point was the 30% salary adjustment, given the normal max was 10%. She said she would write a justification request on my behalf and push the issue with HR. She asked if I could give her more time to work on this, and if it didn't pan out by the time my two-week notice was up, she would certainly understand me leaving. I thanked her and told her of course, without a doubt, I could give her more time. I was overjoyed at this prospect, as I really didn't want to leave Baylor, and this position would lay the groundwork and provide a better foundation for medical school – still my main focus.

As I was awaiting to see what Baylor would be able to do, a call from the Clinical Research Office at UT Southwestern came in. They wanted to interview me for a Research Study Coordinator position. In this role, I would be seeing patients, coordinating trials, and managing protocols to ensure they were followed correctly. I would have a great deal of interaction with the patients and doctors, and the focus would be in BMT HemMalig. This was identical to the position that was in the process of being created at Baylor – just the titles were different. During the interview, I was upfront with them, explaining when I submitted my resignation to Baylor, they offered me a position as a Clinical Research Coordinator and the logistics were still being worked out. Additionally, I explained I also had received a recent offer from US Oncology I was also contemplating. I felt extremely indebted to Baylor at this point. They were pulling out all the stops to not only change the administrative policy in order to create a position I would fit into, but they were also trying to match the offer I had received from US Oncology. I explained to UT Southwestern, it would take quite a bit to pull me from Baylor at this point, and threw out a salary figure I knew would be difficult for them to meet. Their interviewers didn't seem shaken at all at the figure I told them and even said, "Okay." They asked how important the "title" was to me, as all of their Clinical Research Coordinators were nurses, so my title would be Research Study Coordinator. I told them they could call me the "window cleaner" if need be. I didn't really care, a title was just a name. They then said they wanted me to meet the rest of the team I would be working with and toured me around the office. I felt extremely confident leaving the interview. I was on cloud 9. I now had an offer from US Oncology, one in the works from Baylor, and now quite possibly an offer from UT Southwestern, and I knew no matter which avenue I took, I would be overwhelmingly overjoyed.

Never in my wildest imagination at Tech, or anywhere else, did I ever think I would have three different institutions to choose from, with which to work at, in the field of Cancer Research, yet here I was facing this possibility. Words to explain how I felt at the time are impossible to come by. In less than a week from the UT Southwestern interview, both the Baylor position as well as the UT Southwestern one came through. Baylor ended up matching US Oncology's offer and UT Southwestern came a little under what I was asking. It was a pretty easy decision for me at that point, but then Dr. Agura, the Director of the Transplant Program at Baylor, threw me a curve ball. He said a pharmaceutical company had a research position they were funding that was paying six figures and if I wanted it, it was mine. The position entailed me traveling across the US to different BMT centers reviewing patient records, specifically, assays looking at molecular abnormalities in acute leukemia. This information would be compiled into a database used to analyze which abnormalities were common and which were unique.

Purely speculating here, but I believe the pharmaceutical company was trying to determine if there were certain abnormalities that were more rare or common in certain cases of acute leukemia in order to determine the feasibility of generating a "standard" test that could look for these abnormalities in leukemia patients. Beyond that I didn't really have much more information at the time. The money they were offering was very attractive. However, it was explained to me this was a contract position funded by a grant. The grant was guaranteed for a year, but it had the potential to extend closer to three to five years. The other catch – it wouldn't start for a couple months. Although a bit intriguing, and the money sounded good, this opportunity, just had with it too many uncertainties, and I wasn't willing to take the risk. Travel would be difficult as I was still taking classes – remember no gaps in education. Additionally, I couldn't afford to be out of a job if the guarantee turned out to be less than a guarantee. Only a few lose ends to tie up now – call UT Southwestern to decline their offer, but thank them profusely for the opportunity, as you never know when paths may cross again, call US Oncology and explain to them unfortunately I would have to rescind my acceptance of the offer, as Baylor had matched theirs, and that's exactly what I did.

Everything was going great now, my health was good, job had just gotten better, and now I was just waiting for interview requests from the med schools I had applied to, as this was about the time when interviews should start occurring. I was much like a child waiting for a birthday card from the grandparents with money in it. I anxiously, feverishly, checked the mailbox each day, and just as I was beginning to wonder if perhaps the schools somehow had an incorrect address for me – bam – my first letter came. I was overwhelmed with excitement. This was it, and I couldn't wait to open the letter. My excitement was soon replaced by much despair, as I read my first rejection letter. Although, devastated at this point, it was short lived, because I had realized I had applied to 24 schools and surely I would receive some rejection letters in the mix. I only needed one med school to bite, just one interview and I'd be golden. A few more weeks went by and about 20 letters later, I was quickly realizing this wasn't going to be happening this time around and knew I would be re-applying and sitting for the MCAT again. This time though would be different. I would be even more prepared. I knew what to expect from the MCAT now, and I had finished all of my pre-med courses at this point.

The MCAT was only offered twice a year, so I had some time before it would be time to sit for it again. During this time, work was my primary focus, and it was great. I was really enjoying it and it didn't feel like a job at all. Working with patients – patients that were facing the same things I was facing a few years earlier – gave me more fulfillment than I ever could have imagined. Even though at this point, I wasn't a doctor, I felt I was as close as I could be without going to medical school, if that's even possible. Of course, this was only with respect to the very limited, yet specialized, field I was working in. This feeling only further solidified my interest in med school and caused me to push even harder toward that goal.

About six months had gone by now and I was not only coordinating patients on clinical trials, but I was asked to sit on a design team charged with the writing of an Institutional Sponsor Study (IST). This study was looking at utilizing a novel transplant conditioning regimen that was less toxic but just as effective as conventional current transplant conditioning regimens. From study concept to implementation and opening the study for patient accrual, took about a year total and proved vital experience and education, which I thoroughly enjoyed.

Meanwhile, in addition to assisting with the design and developing of this IST, I was managing about eight of our 15 active studies at the time and was responsible for about 35 patients on the studies I was coordinating. Now when I say responsible, I'm not referring to "medical responsibility" as I wasn't a physician, but I worked closely with the doctors and patients to ensure study protocols were followed correctly, patients were dosed accordingly, and safety of the patient was always paramount. Coordinating these trials not only gave me great experience with the disease I was transplanted for, AML, but it also provided great exposure and education regarding all the other hematologic malignancies. This experience proved invaluable and would surely assist in propelling me further towards med school.

MCAT #2 was now upon me. I felt better prepared for it this time around. I had taken many practice tests, read through my MCAT Prep books from the Kaplan Prep Course I took last time, and knew what to expect this time. Additionally, although I was working more now, I had completed all my pre-med courses and was able to solely focus on the MCAT. My score proved this to be true, improving from a 19 to a 21 this time. Yep that's right, after all the prep I had taken, focus I had put in, and practice I had put in, a 21 is what I had to show for it. A far, almost humorous cry, from what I needed. I say humorous now, but I assure you nothing was humorous at the time. It was as if destiny was slapping me in face, telling me to wake up. Snap out of it. Quit trying to develop a reason for why I got leukemia. Still I couldn't, wouldn't give up.

Pursuing med school to become a transplant physician, helping those patients facing the same fears, doubts, and uncertainties I faced, had to be the reason I got sick. I was just being tested. I knew if I took the MCAT one more time, but not let as much time pass between this one and the next, I was sure to do better. This time around – third time I remind you, I added some additional preparatory items to my MCAT prep.

I downloaded some MP3's that focused not so much on "how to take the MCAT" like the Kaplan Course taught. This set of preparation materials focused on intuitively applying the knowledge I had learned in the pre-med school courses to the MCAT questions. Focusing more on what's being asked rather than how to answer the question. At this point, I went ahead and started applying to the med schools, as I could have my MCAT scores sent after my application. I was sure this time it would be closer to 30, and that score, given my personal experience, my work experience, several publications I had written, and numerous letters of recommendation I had received, I was sure to, at the very least, receive one interview. Third time's a charm, as they say, and after I finished the MCAT, I felt more confident this time around than I had the prior two times before.

Applying this time around was a little more difficult than last time. I needed to change up some of my answers, so it didn't look as if I had just copy and pasted them from my prior application. I didn't apply to as many schools this time around either, only about half as many. I applied to the eight med schools in Texas and two out of state – Johns Hopkins and Rosalind Franklin. These two out-of-state med schools really seem to pride themselves on looking at the applicant as a whole, focusing on more than GPA and MCAT score, which I definitely needed given mine.

The other thing that helps with applying to med school is having the backing of a University Committee affiliated with the pre-med program. Essentially, they are vouching for your ability to handle the rigors of med school. Now during my first round of applying to med school, I was taking pre-med courses at UTD and was fortunate to have the backing of their Health Professions Advising Committee (HPAC). In order to use this committee, you had to maintain a certain GPA and meet with advisors from time to time. The committee would serve as a central shipping station for your applications, provide letters of recommendation from two faculty members, write a committee letter on your behalf, and provide "mock" interviews.

Given the huge hurdles I needed to overcome with my latest MCAT score, I felt a backing from the HPAC committee would help me more than ever at this time. The issue with this at this point was, although I was enrolled in the University, I wasn't currently enrolled in class, so I needed to talk with the now "new" committee director, to see if they would assist me again. After getting the meeting set up, I couldn't believe my luck when I walked in to meet the new director. There in the chair sat the former Director of Admissions at UT Southwestern Medical School, the same person I met with all those years earlier when I first started this journey – Dr. Write.

We talked a bit and got reacquainted. He said he was glad I was still pursuing med school. He said he had left UT Southwestern the year prior to when I had first applied to med school. We talked for about an hour and he gave me some great advice and some things to consider. He asked if I had ever given any thought to perhaps looking at one of the foreign med schools. He said there are some in the Caribbean that are 90% American students in my same situation. The admissions standards aren't quite as stiff, and they really do consider more than just GPA and MCAT score. He said the program is four years and when complete, the students transfer to the US for residency programs. They take the same boards, and when it's all said in done, they are licensed to practice medicine in the US, afforded the same rites, duties, and privileges as those students who attended med school in the US. There's no difference. I told him I'd give it some thought and then asked what he thought my chances were of getting them to write me a letter of recommendation, although I wasn't currently enrolled there. He said he wasn't sure, but would discuss it with the committee and see what, if anything he could do.

He contacted me the next day, explaining unfortunately, after discussing with some of his colleagues, they weren't going to be able to write me a letter of recommendation. He further explained they felt it wouldn't be fair to the other students; however, he did say they agreed they would offer to be my central shipping center for my med school applications, which I appreciated. He wished me luck and again told me to consider the foreign med school route and to keep him posted on my progress.

My MCAT scores, now resulted, had been automatically forwarded to the med schools I had applied to this time around. When I saw the results, I knew, unequivocally, I'd be receiving all rejection letters again. My worse score yet was achieved this time with an emphatic 18. The dream of med school was slowly being eroded as each crashing wave of reality crashed and carried pieces of it back out to sea. I was floored, lost, and confused. Getting a rejection letter this time wasn't good enough though. I wanted a reason dammit. I wanted to know what was wrong with my application. Sure, my GPA and MCAT scores were far lower than the lowest of the other applicants, but shouldn't that show balls though? Show tenacity, persistence, determination? I had glowing letters of recommendations from physicians I worked with and from professors I studied under. I had been published in several medical journals. Hell, I worked in cancer research for God's sake. What's more, as a cancer survivor going through the diagnosis and treatment of acute leukemia, including bone marrow transplantation, I offered a unique perspective most doctors couldn't provide. I essentially had everything but GPA and MCAT score, and med schools look at the whole student, right? Right?

I began putting these questions to the med schools I had received rejection letters from, demanding an explanation. I mean I couldn't even score an interview. I cited how in each of their respective admissions requirements, it is listed how the applicant as a whole is considered, but clearly, I felt this was merely a farce. Penning my frustration down to the med schools resulted in me receiving a few "staple form" letters stating how I was welcomed to reapply again once my MCAT and GPA had improved, only adding to my frustration. Mostly I received no reply at all. Two schools though stood out during this time of "frustration airing" – UT Southwestern and Johns Hopkins.

UT Southwestern personally responded to my inquiry, but their response only added fuel to the fire. The new Director of Admissions emailed me, explaining most likely I would never get into their med school given my GPA and MCAT score. He explained those scores statistically demonstrate who can and who cannot handle the rigors of med school. I explained it's ridiculous to allow one standardized test, and, in my case, the culmination of grades over the course of 10+ years, to make that determination, without even interviewing me. He pressed on, indicating past statistics demonstrated that in fact was the case. He interjected stating there are standardized tests throughout med school, which would also prove difficult for me if I weren't a good test taker. I just wanted a chance I explained, to which he indicated UT Southwestern, unfortunately, wouldn't be able to give me that chance, as I was just too big a risk for them.

Similarly, I was contacted by Johns Hopkins. I had stepped away from my desk to go see a patient and upon my return, I noticed I had a voicemail. It was from the Associate Dean of Admissions wanting to discuss my pursuit of med school. I couldn't believe I was listening to a message from the Associate Dean of Admissions at Johns Hopkins. Clearly my email bathed in frustration had reached them. The fact the Associate Dean took time out of her day to reach out to me personally, had me buzzing with cautious optimism. Yes, I was at work and I had plenty of things to do, but I dropped everything I was doing, texted Dr. Berryman relaying Hopkins wanted to talk with me, and rushed to call her back. We talked for about an hour – even Dr. Berryman talked to her. She mentioned she wished she would have met me years earlier, before I had embarked on this journey. She explained she could have better advised me on how I could have bettered my chances of acceptance into medical school. Rather than just merely taking the pre-med courses, it would have been better for me to get a post-bachelorette degree in Biology or Bio-Chem. She said although I had taken the pre-med courses and done fairly well in them, my actual degree, the "Bachelor's" I received from Tech, was the degree tied to my GPA and that GPA was a 2.1.

She also mentioned it is absolutely true med schools look at the applicant as a whole, especially at John's Hopkins, but the 2.1 GPA that was tied to my Bachelor's was just too difficult to overcome, or have overlooked, given my low MCAT score, without another degree to fall on. She also asked if I had given any thought to foreign medical schools and suggested if that wasn't an option to go back and start again from scratch to obtain a post-bachelorette degree. If I did well with that degree, strengthened my MCAT scores, then perhaps, I'd have a better chance. She pressed on stating she knew this was a daunting task given how much effort I had already put into it, but stressed she believed it was the only way and even still it wasn't a guarantee.

At this point, I took everything in and was quite shaken. I was second guessing myself and questioning if this was really what I was supposed to be doing. All the signs were saying otherwise. I had taken the MCAT now three times, applied to medical school twice, spent close to 30K with all the classes, application fees, MCAT tests, and preparation materials. What did I really have to show for it at this point? I really had a great deal to think about now. Little did I know at this time, as I have often found during this snap shot of my life, things were already slowly at work, making this decision for me, shifting my focus yet again.

Our BMT research program was growing and I was becoming more and more focused on work and the patients I was working with on the studies I was coordinating. Honestly, I was too busy to think about med school right now. I had recently co-authored an abstract, published in Blood, reviewing recent results of a clinical trial I was not only coordinating patients on, but also helped with the design of. The abstract had been selected for presentation at one of the national conferences on hematologic malignancies, and the poster accompanying the abstract that I'd be presenting, highlighted our results. This would be my fourth meeting and fifth time to present, but something was different about this meeting. Maybe because at this meeting, I felt I was at a crossroads. I wasn't sure what to do regarding my faltering attempt at pursuing med school up to this point.

About mid-way through the meeting though, I had made my decision. My passion was med school. Attending this meeting and hearing of all the novel cutting edge research that was currently going on and seeing what type of potential treatment modalities lie ahead, reinvigorated me in my med school aspirations. I decided I would once again make one final attempt and much like the trip to Ohio will always hold a special place in my heart, this trip would as well, but of course for different reasons. This was my "decision trip," the trip when my path became firmly set.

I had already decided, far before it was even suggested to me twice now, attending a foreign med school wasn't going to work. Elisse was now working as an attorney building her career and I wasn't going to ask her to uproot everything while I go chase this dream overseas. Going the post-bachelorette degree route wasn't an option either. I had already come this far, and wasn't about to start over.

My plan was to take the MCAT one last time, just once more. It had now been three years since I first took the MCAT, so my first score, 19, would not be included in my application this time, as they only went back three years when looking at scores. While prepping for the MCAT this final time, I would take Anatomy and Physiology – remember no gaps in education. Anatomy and Physiology was another class I was highly interested in taking, so I anticipated doing well in it. When I returned home from this meeting, I would begin preparations for this one last attempt.

The week-long meeting was coming to a close. While on the phone with Elisse on one of the final evenings, I was sharing some of the interesting research coming down the pike. Now when I start to talk about this, I suspect it sounds as interesting to her as it does when she discusses lawyering with me. Nonetheless, I can sometimes get a bit too excited and ramble a bit I suppose.

For the most part Elisse is patient with me and, at the very least, pretends to listen. This evening though, I could tell I didn't have her 100% focus, which was confirmed when she interjected with some information of her own. No, she wasn't pregnant, and if she was, that would be alarming information for me. I was sterile remember, due to chemo and radiation. Along those lines; however, it did have to do with a child. She mentioned when I returned that we would be babysitting a little boy, which I was fine with. How hard could it be, as I've babysat before. No biggie. Then she dropped the bomb on me asking what I thought about maybe adopting him. What? Adopting? Who? What? I totally didn't see that coming and was completely caught off guard. Adoption itself wasn't the issue. We had talked extensively about adoption and how we were going to have a family someday. We had previously discussed starting this process two or so years down the road. Remember we had sperm banked all those years earlier – roughly eight years earlier now at this point, around the time I was starting chemo. We knew, given my limited supply, only six vials, it wasn't a sure thing. We had already decided we wanted to adopt first, given the uncertainty of success with non-conventional methods. Through adoption, if we were unsuccessful in our attempts with IUI or IVF, then we would have already been blessed with a child, so the loss would be far less difficult to cope with. But this was supposed to start two years down the road, not now, and when Elisse dropped this bomb on me, it was this timing I was caught off guard with.

I was highly against doing this now and had lots of questions. I didn't know what to think or how to process, being the next two years would be upon us in two days now. She said he was between four and five years old, had blond hair and blue eyes. His mom had him when she was 17 and initially thought she could raise him, with the help of friends and her mom. Reality for the mom quickly set in and she realized her view of reality was not "real" reality. Elisse continued, explaining her situation became more difficult when she had child #2 less than a year after child #1. She had no stable job. She was between boyfriends. She was between homes. I felt for the mom and the situation she was in and the children, but ultimately, I was deadset against it. I said, "Four or five? That's way too old and at that age kids are already screwed up, especially if they had been passed around from mom's friends to friends and back and forth." I wanted to wait and said we just need to stick to our plan. We can look at adoption in a couple of years, when we're both further along, like we had originally discussed. She pushed on explaining we'll at least meet him, as she already committed us to babysitting him this coming weekend. Whatever. I told her why even ask my opinion if it's already been made for me? She said it's just one weekend and we'll see how it goes.

I asked how all this played out with our names getting thrown in the mix. Elisse explained that her boss, Donald and his wife Hillary, ran a maternity home for young mothers and one of her girls realized she wasn't able to raise him, nor was she ready to be a mom, both financially and emotionally. She was looking to place him with a family through adoption. Donald and Hillary knew our situation about wanting to adopt at some time down the road and asked if we'd be interested in assisting with fostering and caring for him on weekends and when they were out of town.

Again, I stressed four or five is just too old and felt if we went down this path now, I thought we would be opening ourselves up to lot of difficulty and disappointment. I mean, we knew nothing about this kid. Who knew what he had been exposed to with being passed around back and forth without any stability or structure over the course of his lifetime. It had the potential to be a mistake we would not be able to undo and would have to face it for the rest of our lives.

Now, Elisse is an attorney, and very skilled at the art of arguing or discussing as I like to call it. She simply won the argument/discussion by explaining it would be a crazy mistake, not to at least consider the opportunity. No risk, no reward. She knew as an attorney and seeing first hand, adoption can be a long drawn out highly emotional process and for this to just fall in our laps at this time had to be sent from above. She continued, adding, who knows what will be two years from now. Being that all the things I was certain to go one way, actually ended up going a completely opposite way, I couldn't argue this and relented.

She was right and I agreed we'd keep him over the weekend, which I explained will be even more interesting being my parents were coming up and would undoubtedly have some questions.

The night before I had been at a conference discussing cutting edge research in hematologic malignancies, and now we were on our way to meet and pick up a child we had never seen before, but had the possibility of becoming our son – crazy and not sure if I was ready for this change. When we met him, I was surprised at how small he was and what little vocabulary he had. Also, his gait was very unstable and he seemed highly uncoordinated, clumsy, and all over the place. Nonetheless, he was definitely adorable and full of energy. His name was Landon. I was excited after meeting him, and became even more so, when Elisse leaned over to tell me she got the age wrong. He was actually 1.5 years old. I figured that was the case as he certainly didn't sound, act, or move like he was almost five.

We took Landon back home with us and were quickly reminded we were very experienced parents of "quadrupeds," but severely lacking in that regard with "bipeds." We had no idea what to feed him. Surprisingly, his limited vocabulary was all that we needed to help us in that regard. Landon's vocabulary at that point consisted of three words – "eat eat," "McDonald's," and "funf fries." In that instant, not only did we know what we could feed him, but we also learned what his diet primarily consisted of up to that point. We opted for a local sit down restaurant close to our home. We knew he was pleased when he exclaimed "funf fries, funf fries" with a grin from ear to ear. He ate them all, and even ate all his chicken strips as well. It didn't take long for me to switch my opinion on adoption now rather than later, less than an hour. We were hooked and ready jump on board.

My parents fell in love with Landon right off the bat as well. And intelligence. It was unbelievable to see just how smart he was, even with his limited vocabulary. In no time, he was calling me 'papa' and Elisse 'mama.' Although fully on board, we still had to remain somewhat guarded at this time. We knew things were still up in the air and great deal of legal issues had to be worked out before we were even close to adoption. Additionally, we knew at any time, the mom could always change her mind, so this was a tricky time for us.

While waiting on the adoption process and all things that entailed, I had begun working towards med school again. I had begun the Anatomy and Physiology (A&P) class and was studying at night, as we had Landon on the weekends. We were building our relationship and becoming a family, although we tried to remain guarded. Since he didn't really have any male role models in his life, Landon attached superfast to me – which would prove vital in the near future. A&P was going generally well. I was struggling a bit, but had a "B" in the class, so I was pleased. Work was also going well and everyone was excited and praying for Elisse and I as we embarked on this new chapter. My final was coming up for my class and after it was over, I was extremely glad to be done with school for a while – then and there it hit me. Did I really want to go to med school?

Even if by some miracle, and believe me, I knew I had already been the recipient of plenty up to now, I got in, the program I wanted would take a total of nine years to complete. Did I really want to spend these early years studying all the time rather than spending time with our son, should the adoption work out? The answer was an emphatic no. I began to realize for the second time now, I had been given this wonderful second chance at life. Much like the first time I asked what I really wanted to do with this second chance, I realized my focused had now changed again.

I wanted to stop trying to get to a place I may, or may not, ever reach. I wanted to just live the life I had been given. I wanted to travel. To enjoy life. I didn't want to study and take tests and prepare, all to be over 40 when I could finally be done with all the schooling, but then only to be a slave to my patients and practice, that would surely be demanded of me as a transplant physician, should the opportunity present itself. I decided it wasn't fair to myself, nor my wife, nor my future children, be it this one we were trying to adopt or any others that may come our way in the future. I didn't want this anymore. I wanted something far more important and doing it in my "spare time" wasn't enough. The time had come for me to be a dad now – or 'Papa' rather.

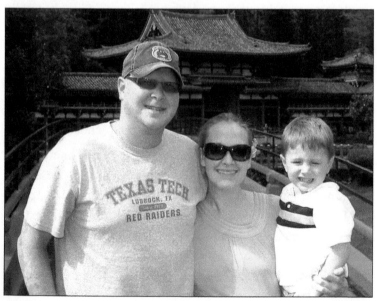

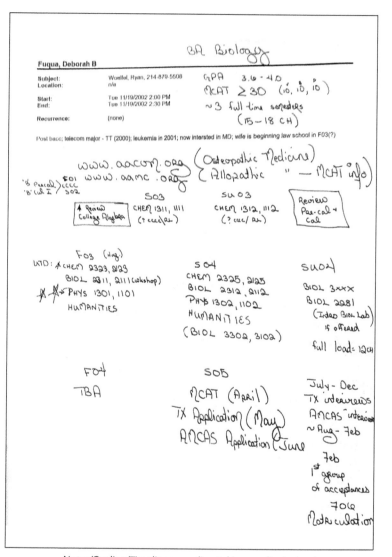

*Notes/Outline/Timeline regarding taking medical school
pre-requisite courses and then applying to medical school*

Progress Note

Robert Brian Berryman, MD
Texas Cancer Center
at Medical City Dallas
7777 Forest Lane, D-220
Dallas, Texas 75230

Patient:	Woelfel, Ryan	MedRecNum:	50093
Dictate:	02/06/03	Visitation:	02/04/03
TScribe:	02/07/03 ndb		

REASON FOR VISIT: AML status post allogeneic related stem cell transplant February 2, 2001.

INTERVAL HISTORY: Mr. Woelfel has no new complaints today. His chronic cutaneous GVHD manifested by vitiligo is unchanged. His energy level is good. He currently is working and getting his master's degree. He is also interested in going back to medical school. He denies any problems related to GVH.

INTERVAL PAST MEDICAL HISTORY: Unchanged.

INTERVAL SOCIAL HISTORY: Unchanged.

INTERVAL FAMILY HISTORY: Unchanged.

CURRENT MEDICATIONS: Bactrim, multivitamins, topical steroids as needed, artificial tears, and vitamin B_{12} complex.

ALLERGIES: None.

REVIEW OF SYSTEMS:
GENERAL: Taking medications as prescribed. Denies fevers, nausea, or weight loss.
SKIN: Positive for vitiligo.
HEENT: Vision unchanged. No headaches, sinus symptoms, hearing problems, sore mouth, or sore throat.
CHEST/LUNGS: No cough, shortness of breath, or sputum production. No catheter site redness or pain.
CARDIOVASCULAR: No chest pains or palpitations.
GASTROINTESTINAL: No nausea, vomiting, abdominal pain, diarrhea, or constipation.
GENITOURINARY: No problems with urination. No genitorectal problems.
NEUROLOGIC: No confusion, tremors, or depression.
MUSCULOSKELETAL: No weakness, arthritis, or trouble walking.
EXTREMITIES: No localized swelling or weakness.
LYMPH NODES: No swollen lymph glands or new or unusual lumps.
ENDOCRINE: No history of diabetes or thyroid disease.

Note from Dr. Brian Berryman after
we had discussed my interest in medical school

Woelfel, Ryan
02/04/03
Page 2

PHYSICAL EXAMINATION:
VITAL SIGNS: Normal. Afebrile.
GENERAL: Healthy-appearing, ambulatory.
SKIN: Positive for vitiligo.
HEENT: Normocephalic. Pupils round and reactive. Sclerae anicteric
Oropharynx without lesions.
NECK: Supple without lymph nodes.
CHEST: Clear to auscultation and percussion.
CATHETER: Catheter site without erythema, tenderness, or drainage.
CARDIOVASCULAR: Without murmurs, rubs, or gallops. Regular rate and
rhythm.
ABDOMEN: Soft without hepatosplenomegaly.
LYMPH NODES: Superficial lymph nodes are not palpable in all areas.
EXTREMITIES: No cyanosis, clubbing, or edema.
NEURO: Nonfocal sensory, motor, cranial nerve, cerebellar, and mental status
testing.

LABORATORY DATA: CBC shows a white count of 6.4, hematocrit 44,
platelets 215,000. His chemistries are unremarkable, including normal liver
function tests.

IMPRESSION: Mr. Woelfel is a 26-year-old white man with a history of acute
myelogenous leukemia status post allogeneic related stem cell transplant.

PROBLEM LIST:
1. AML. The patient is in complete remission with full engraftment and a normal
   CBC.
2. Infectious disease. The patient will continue Bactrim. He will receive his
   14-month vaccinations.
3. GVHD. Clinically stable. We will treat symptomatically with topical steroids
   and artificial tears.

Robert Brian Berryman, MD

*Page 2 of the note from Dr. Brian Berryman after
we had discussed my interest in medical school*

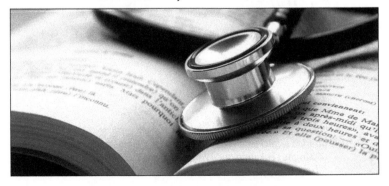

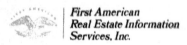

First American
Real Estate Information
Services, Inc.

August 18, 2003

RE: Sponsorship

Ryan Woelfel
First American National Search
8435 N. Stemmons Freeway
Dallas, TX 75247

Dear Ryan,

On behalf of First American and First American Real Estate Tax Service, I am pleased to present you with a check in the amount of $1,000.00 for the Leukemia & Lymphoma Society.

At First American we pride ourselves in giving back to the community and to organizations that help others.

Thank you for giving us the opportunity to support this worthwhile organization

Sincerely,

Rick Holcomb

Donation letter I received on behalf of First American donating
$1000 to the Leukemia and Lymphoma Society. This was money
I was trying to raise while working on "team n' training"

Woelfel, Ryan

From:	Elisse Woelfel/Building Products/Euramax [EWoelfel@amerimaxbp.com]
Sent:	Tuesday, September 14, 2004 11:16 AM
To:	Woelfel, Ryan
Subject:	Baylor

Welcome to Baylor! We look forward to having you join our team. I am forwarding you
instructions for our pre-employment process. Hopefully, it will assist you with a
smooth new hire transition. Please feel free to contact me at any time during the
process if you have questions AT (214) 820-7009.

All employment offers are contingent Upon successful completion of the Background
Check and pre-employment Employee Health Screening.

Background Check/Verification

Due to the nature of our business, Baylor University Medical Center completes a
thorough background check of all new employees. The background check includes:
pre-employment physical, drug screen, employment reference and criminal background
check. Where applicable, license, certification and/or registrations will be
verified as well.

The Supplemental Data form is required documentation that includes your employer
information, contacts, location and dates; licensure and/or certifications, and your
signed authorization for the background check. If you did not complete this form in
your initial interview, please contact Human Resources to request this form. The
Supplemental Data form must be completed in order to initiate the background check
and employment verification.

Welcome letter from Baylor accepting me into the
Blood and Marrow Transplantation Research Program –
I was overjoyed at the prospect of this new journey

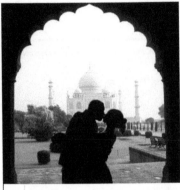

Elisse and I at the Taj Mahal while visiting Lori in India. This is about 4 years post transplant.

Progress Note

Sammons C. Center/Texas Oncology, P A
3535 Worth St   Dallas, TX 75246

Patient: WOELFEL, RYAN G		MR# 467-89-6877		Visit Date	12/13/2004	
Att Phy: ROBERT B BERRYMAN MD		DD. 12/14/2004		DT	12/16/2004 13 59 29	cpw

REASON FOR VISIT: AML, status post allogeneic related peripheral blood stem cell transplant 11/18/2000

INTERVAL HISTORY: Mr. Woelfel who had a transplant at Medical City Dallas. He has been followed there and has recently transferred his care here to Baylor. In addition, he is employed here. He comes in today to clinic for routine followup. He has no complaints today. His post-transplant course has been complicated by chronic graft-versus-host disease. This has been manifested with cutaneous involvement with vitiligo. Otherwise, he has no complaints. He is recovering from an upper respiratory infection and was treated with Levaquin for this. These symptoms have resolved.

INTERVAL PAST MEDICAL HISTORY: Unchanged.

INTERVAL SOCIAL HISTORY: Unchanged.

INTERVAL FAMILY HISTORY: Unchanged.

CURRENT MEDICATIONS:
1. Acyclovir.
2. Multivitamin.
3. Elidel.
4. Protopic.
5. Flaxseed oil.
6. B-complex.

ALLERGIES: None.

REVIEW OF SYSTEMS:
GENERAL: Taking medications as prescribed. Denies fevers, nausea, or weight loss.
SKIN: Positive for vitiligo.
HEENT: Vision unchanged. No headaches, sinus symptoms, hearing problems, sore mouth, or sore throat.
CHEST/LUNGS: No cough, shortness of breath, or sputum production.
CARDIOVASCULAR: No chest pains or palpitations.
GASTROINTESTINAL: No nausea, vomiting, abdominal pain, diarrhea, or constipation.
GENITOURINARY: No problems with urination. No genitorectal problems.
NEUROLOGIC: No confusion, tremors, or depression.
MUSCULOSKELETAL: No weakness, arthritis, or trouble walking.
EXTREMITIES: No localized swelling or weakness.
LYMPH NODES: No swollen lymph glands or new or unusual lumps.

PHYSICAL EXAMINATION:
VITAL SIGNS: Blood pressure 150/95. Pulse 90. Temperature 97.7.
GENERAL: Healthy-appearing, ambulatory.
SKIN: Positive for vitiligo.

WOELFEL, RYAN G
12/13/2004
Page 2 of 2

PHYSICAL EXAMINATION: (continued)
HEENT Normocephalic Pupils round and reactive. Sclerae anicteric. Oropharynx without lesions
NECK Supple without lymph nodes
CHEST Clear to auscultation and percussion.
CARDIOVASCULAR Without murmurs, rubs, or gallops. Regular rate and rhythm.
ABDOMEN Soft without hepatosplenomegaly.
LYMPH NODES Superficial lymph nodes are not palpable in all areas.
EXTREMITIES No cyanosis, clubbing, or edema.
NEURO Nonfocal sensory, motor, cranial nerve, cerebellar, and mental status testing

LABORATORY DATA:
CBC White count 6 9 Hematocrit 46. Platelets 254. Differential: 49 polys; 35 lymphs; 14 monos.
CHEMISTRIES Chemistries and liver function studies are normal.

IMPRESSION/PLAN: The patient is a 28-year-old white gentleman with a history of AML, status post allogeneic transplant

PROBLEMS:
1. AML. The patient is in remission and will be restaged with XY FISH now four years out from his transplant.
2. Infectious disease. No active infections. We will check IgG subclasses and total for recurrent bronchitis. The patient may benefit from intravenous immunoglobulin (IV.G). He also may benefit from Levaquin chronic prophylaxis.
3. Graft-versus-host disease. Continue topical therapy.
4. Hypertension. The patient will keep a blood pressure diary over the next week. He may need an antihypertensive. He is not on any medications associated with this, with the exception possibly of Sudafed, which he took for his upper respiratory infection, although, it has been three days plus since he has taken his last dosage.

Robert Brian Berryman, MD

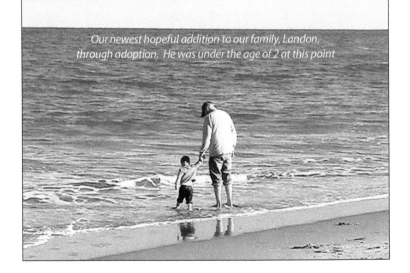

Our newest hopeful addition to our family, Landon, through adoption. He was under the age of 2 at this point

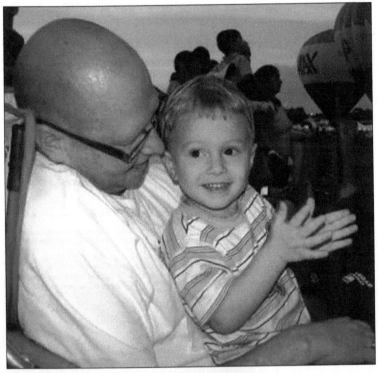

The Plano Balloon Festival

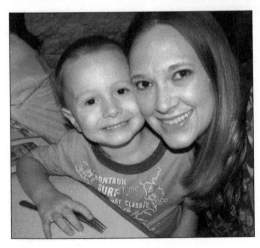

Elisse and Landon – we were definitely hooked and loving the idea of being his parents

Chapter 9: New Family

Really there was no way to prepare me for how much our lives would change as we attempted to embark on this new journey – parenthood. The next few weeks and months would prove to be an emotional rollercoaster for all involved. Although we tried to stay guarded with our emotions and attachment to Landon, it was not possible – we were 100% all in. Each weekend we had him, we all bonded more and more – we were becoming a family.

Donald (Elisse's boss) and Hillary (his wife) had legal custody of Landon, so he was staying at their house. Each Friday night after work, if Hillary didn't bring him to the law firm where Elisse worked, we would go pick him up at their house. This quickly became our routine. On some occasions while Donald and Hillary were heading out of town for the weekend, or on an extended vacation, we would keep him for entire weeks or even longer at a time. This provided great opportunity for us to all bond even more so as a family.

As time went on, this cycle continued to the point when we began to wonder if we were ever going to move forward with adoption. Although, we were happy with any amount of time we were getting to have with Landon, we were beginning to feel as if we were just merely convenient weekend babysitters. Things were stagnant. We had not received any indications of how things were progressing towards the adoption process and all the legalities that accompany it.

We were in a tricky spot as we couldn't push too much, because Donald was Elisse's boss, and they had legal custody of him. Additionally, Hillary, who seemed to control most things, was attached to Landon as well, and they had adopted another child in a similar situation. We had to be careful, as we didn't want her to stop or slow our progress. We talked with the biological mother, Jordy, on a few occasions, but she always seemed to be unsure, or on the fence with what she wanted to do. She was up for adoption, and liked us to be the adopted parents, but it was the "when" that she was on the fence about, as her mother was still unsure. On one occasion, in fact, Jordy was asked to sign parental termination rights, to which she agreed, but then was a no-show. Elisse and I were in the picture, but kind of from a distance, with Donald and Hillary keeping us updated. We were really getting concerned, as we kept hearing different stories, and weren't sure if the outcome was going to be in our favor.

Hearing multiple different stories and this back and forth continued. We would hear from Jordy that all was good to go and her mother, Shelby, wanted to meet us. Then, immediately, Hillary would say, it was Shelby that was the problem and holding things up. Hillary quite bluntly indicated, Shelby had no personal interest in him, but didn't want him to be adopted out. She felt he was blood and needed to be raised by blood relatives. She had her three kids early on in a similar situation and felt if she could do it, then Jordy should be able to as well. From the things we heard regarding Shelby, we definitely were not fans and pretty judgmental of her.

Our opinion of her remained pretty dismal until we met her that is. Jordy had invited us to meet Shelby at Landon's two year old birthday party. His younger half-sister (child #2), would also be there, as it was her one year old birthday party. Remember, Landon and his half-sister were just 364 days apart. Elisse and I were excited to see Landon again, but also nervous to be meeting Shelby, given our impression of her. Sure enough, this was when we began to see Shelby for who and what she really was – a great person who truly cared and wanted what was best for Landon. The picture of her that had been painted by Hillary couldn't have been further from the truth. We talked with her for about an hour or so. We learned and could see first-hand she truly did care for him, but wanted to be a grandmother, which was understandable. She had been a parent already, three times over with her own children. She definitely wanted a relationship with him, but could not or would not raise him. We told her we wanted the same thing as her and we were wanting an open adoption. We would let and encourage her to be as involved or as uninvolved as she wanted. This was the same way we approached Jordy, as we felt he could never have too many people around loving him.

After our meeting, Elisse and I were now convinced it wasn't Shelby at all holding things up, she just didn't fully understand what the process was or what was going on. Shelby said she would get calls from Hillary asking her if she wanted to see him, or visit with him, with no notice at all. When Shelby would try to reschedule a time that would work for her, often times Hillary would just hang up on her. We could easily see we weren't getting the whole story from Hillary, which again concerned us.

It had already been five months since we met Landon, and we didn't feel any closer to adopting him now than we did in the beginning. We turned up the heat a bit more and began to apply some more pressure. We wanted to know when we were moving forward, when Jordy would be signing parental rights termination papers. We had no way to know what progress was being made, as we had to rely on Donald to keep us updated. He assured us he was working on it and things were moving in the right direction. He was confident things would work out for us, he just needed a bit more time. This cycle continued for few more weeks, then out of nowhere, one day, it all abruptly came to an end.

Elisse had asked Hillary if we were getting Landon for the weekend and she said not this weekend for some reason or another. Elisse and I were disappointed, as we had been accustomed to having him on the weekends, but our hands were tied at this point. Even though most weekends, we got him, there were some weekends – few and far between – when we didn't, and just figured this was one of those times.

Elisse had made some plans to go out with some friends the next night, and less than a half hour before it was time for her to go, Hillary called asking if we wanted to come get Landon for the weekend. Elisse reminded Hillary, she had already told us we wouldn't be getting him this weekend, and mentioned she was on her way out the door to meet some friends. Elisse asked Hillary if anything was wrong, and then out of nowhere, Hillary started shouting at Elisse, saying maybe she wasn't fit to be a mother after all and abruptly hung up the phone.

Elisse, in tears, called me telling me what had just happened. I asked her to call Hillary back and find out what's wrong and what just happened here. Elisse explained she had already tried several times but was just getting her voice mail. What the hell just happened? What did we do? Did we do something to piss her off? We were totally lost and at this point, highly concerned.

We were supposed to come get him the next day, but now we were unsure if that was now off the table because of what just transpired. Both Elisse and I each called both Donald and Hillary repeatedly to no avail – straight to voicemail every time.

That weekend was one of the longest ones we had ever experienced thus far, but it didn't get any better, as all we heard Monday from Donald was to just give Hillary some time and lay low. What? Lay low? Give her some time? What the hell, here we were fully attached to Landon and fully committed to doing whatever it took, by any means necessary to have him, and now we're being told by the very people who are supposed to be helping us to "lay low," to "back off" and "be patient." Are you kidding me? This silent treatment went on for a little over a month with no news regarding Landon, or when we could see him again.

Anytime we brought it up, we were told the same lines – just back off a bit and give it some time, blah, blah, blah. I was so livid and was strongly contemplating picking him up at his daycare and splitting to Mexico to start over. Luckily, we never had to find out how much of that was emotions talking vs. a real possibility. Thankfully by the grace of God and Landon's bond to us and his constant crying because he missed us and wanted to see us again, Hillary finally relented. She called us asking if we would like to come get him for the weekend, and without hesitation, we were on our way.

It was as if no time had passed at all, and I was determined to never get in that situation again. We were going to be kissing ass for as long as it took. Accept all the blame given to us for whatever issue there was and do whatever possible to keep Hillary happy. Given the emotional roller coaster we just experienced, we knew time was of the essence and immediately started the ball rolling, at least as much as we could. Meanwhile, Shelby had contacted Jordy, expressing her wishes and explained that she needed to do the right thing and sign the termination papers so things could start going in the right direction. Shortly thereafter, that's exactly what happened, and the very next step we needed to do was find a daycare close to us that we could transition him to.

We stumbled upon a daycare that actually shared the same parking lot as Elisse's law firm. We checked it out and couldn't believe our luck. The daycare was a Christian-based daycare and it was a Chinese one as well. We thought the Chinese was icing on the cake. We figured by the time Landon was in middle school, Spanish would be a requirement like math and science, meaning he would already be learning Spanish. We wanted to give him an edge, so Chinese was a great language for him to learn, and being that he was two, it was the perfect time for him to start.

We told Donald and Hillary about the daycare and asked if they thought we could move him to the daycare now rather than later, as things were beginning to move in the right direction. They agreed, said they were happy things seemed to be working out, and even offered to pay the first month's cost and upfront deposit. Of course, we took them up on their offer, although the offer never really materialized, but that was a minor inconvenience at this point. We were just happy things were finally progressing.

You may wonder about the biological father as I haven't mentioned anything of him – that's basically because he's really unmentionable in all this. Elisse met with him once to see if he would be willing to terminate his parental rights, to which he inquired if that would also terminate any financial responsibility he might have, and he agreed and terminated his parental rights. Elisse performed the other necessary legalities and checked the paternal registry, to make sure there were no loose ends, and we were good to go from his standpoint.

All the chips were now falling into place. Our home study had been completed and our hearing had been set. Here we were ready to adopt this wonderful boy, Landon, who was brought into our lives just seven months earlier. Our hearing had been set for September 9, 2009, and that was the day Elisse and I went from becoming just a couple to a family. After the adoption hearing, we all went out to celebrate and it was a full house. My parents, Elisse's parents, Jordy, Shelby, Landon's half-sister and her paternal grandparents (who had adopted her at the same hearing), and even Donald and Hillary all went to the same place to eat where we ate the first night we babysat Landon seven months earlier, and by chance, we even got the same waitress we had that night as well.

Perhaps you noticed I mentioned his half-sister, Harley, had also been adopted by her paternal grandparents at the same hearing. After Landon was born, Jordy had met someone else and after sometime, they together felt they could raise a child of their own and gave it a shot. A short nine months later, Harley was born. I think having two kids now, being 19, and no real way to support them, was the impetus to placing Landon with adoption – thankfully for us.

Fast-forward now to this point in time and I think the realization occurred that it would also be difficult raising Harley for the same reasons, so they decided to place her up for adoption as well. You might wonder why we didn't try to keep them together, but we did. We asked about adopting Harley as well, but the paternal grandparents wanted nothing to do with that. They said blood would raise blood, so we accepted their decision and moved on.

Once the celebration was over and we had gotten home, I got the dollar bill that I took as a sign eight years earlier that we would have children one day and framed it and hung it on the wall. Having Landon on the weekends actually provided a smooth transition, where everything seemed normal and natural. There were no rough patches and everything went smoothly. We left it up to Jordy and Shelby as to when they wanted to come visit and never denied or pushed any sort of relationship on their parts. When they did get together, everything went smooth and again everything seemed as this was always meant to be, which made it easy for all involved.

Life was great. We were now a family, living life and enjoying life. I was happy with my decision to not attempt med school again. I was satisfied with the field I was working in and felt fulfilled. I was still working on cutting edge research in the field that saved my life, and although I wasn't doing so as a doctor, I still worked closely with them, was learning a great deal, and felt it was as close as I was going to be able to get and that was fine. I still loved my job, and it was going good, but there were some noticeable changes going on – new leadership, among other things. It seemed to me the place I thoroughly enjoyed working at, was now becoming more business and revenue focused rather than research focused. This wasn't so much true of the doctors, nurses, and staff I worked with, but more so with the administration. It seemed to me the focus now was to grow the program by accepting any study that came our way, rather than looking closely at what the study was actually for. Something Dr. Fay (the doctor that started the transplant program at Baylor) said regarding this that has always stuck with me was, "...it's better to focus on three, four, or five studies we can really learn something from or develop something novel with, rather than to do 15 or 20 studies no one really has an interest in, or the time to focus on given the large patient load...," and I wholeheartedly agreed.

I had been working in a research capacity at Baylor now for roughly seven years and this gradual shift of the focus of research under this new administration in our department, at least from my perspective, wasn't the only issue I was having. I began having recruiters contact me, telling me I was way underpaid and that I should be making about 30% more given the experience I had now developed over the course of my employment. Remember I was hearing this from several recruiters, and of course I felt I was underpaid – don't we all, but I had no idea just how underpaid I was. I didn't want to leave Baylor, as I felt eternally indebted to the transplant physicians and the people who helped me get in this field and taught me so much. At the same time though, I felt a discussion was at the very least warranted.

My angle was simple – I worked on a team with research nurses and although I was not a nurse, our jobs were identical in every aspect but salary. I was making roughly half of what the nurses were, for the simple fact I wasn't a nurse. Not to take anything away from nurses. I have the utmost respect for them. Remember, I was also a patient and know how crucial they are. The simple fact was the research nurses I worked with did not perform "traditional 'floor' nursing" duties. The clinic nurses did those things. The research nurses I worked with did the exact same duties I did; yet again they were paid twice as much. Some of the nurses had only associate degrees in nursing. Yes, they were still RN's, but I had a Bachelor's degree, so more education, and I had more "research" experience. That was neither here nor there, as my main argument was we were performing the same task, yet there was a huge unjustifiable compensation disparity.

I eventually met with the administrators, asking not to be paid like our nurses, but to just be paid more comparable to them. Their response, "...if you want to be paid like a nurse... go to nursing school...." This absolutely floored me. I was handling more studies than our nurses, covering other disease department's studies, and was fielding questions from some of the very nurses that were making twice as much as I was. It wasn't long before I started rethinking my loyalty to the place that got me started; however, I felt I was not being treated very loyally either, at least not by the new administration.

Although work life was beginning to get a bit more cumbersome as my dissatisfaction grew, home life was getting more excited. Landon was now four years old and we were looking into using all that powerful super-sperm we had been banking and paying for so long. I had done enough research to know that in the process of thawing and washing the sperm, over 50% would be lost. This meant our best chance was to couple any existing sperm I currently had, with what we had frozen 12 years earlier. No problem, except radiation + chemo = sterility, so my current supply was nada, zilch, zero. With this being the case, our supply was limited only to the six frozen vials we had banked. We were wanting to go the conventional non-conventional route of intrauterine implantation (IUI), but in the back of our minds, Elisse and I both knew in-vitro fertilization (IVF) was an option. We were hoping to avoid that option if at all possible, not only due to the cost associated with it, but also because of the insurmountable decision concerning which embryos to keep and what to do with the ones we didn't keep, in the event of multiples – a decision neither of us wanted to make.

We had our first consultation, and I must admit, I was a bit nervous, given the research I had already done and the limited supply we had. We brought along my sperm processing/banking records from 12 years prior, and when the doctor took a look at them, all of our fears disappeared. The doctor explained to us the target number of sperm they are hoping to see in collected samples used for IUI was 10-20 million. My two deposits had close to 150 million each, so we had roughly 300 million sperm to work with. Powerful super sperm? Definitely. I must say I'm pretty proud of that number and the studness-ness it confirms.

We were elated. What this meant was we didn't have to worry about my current supply, or lack thereof. Even with the loss associated with post processing and thawing, we would still have plenty to work with and then some. The next step was to get Elisse checked out and she checked out perfectly with no issues whatsoever. Now another waiting game had begun. We needed to wait for Elisse to ovulate and then rush to the doctor's office for the procedure.

I never thought I would be so excited to hear my wife was ovulating, but that was definitely the case when she told me, and immediately we headed up to the doctor's office for the procedure. The procedure went well, was relatively uneventful, not too romantic, and definitely not as much fun as the conventional method of baby making is. After the thaw and processing, we had the amount needed for the procedure in one vial, leaving us with five more to work with if need be. We returned home to wait some more with our fingers crossed it would take and we'd be pregnant soon. We waited and waited and waited some more and then realized this first attempt didn't take. We were both a little upset; however, not too much so, as we still had five more shots. We also had Landon, the best son in the world, so we were okay at this point.

At our next doctor's appointment, we inquired about methods that could potentially improve our chances. She mentioned we could use two vials this time and we could self-administer a shot that would trigger Elisse's ovulation, so we could be sure the procedure was performed at the optimal time-point in the ovulation cycle. We agreed and felt this would be our best chance and again it was a waiting game until Elisse began to cycle again.

As my home family life was becoming more and more exciting, it was becoming more and more apparent to me that my work life was beginning to take a nose dive. I thoroughly enjoyed working with the doctors I worked with as well as the people I worked with. The problem I was having was with the administration, and the direction I felt the research department was headed. I felt it was quickly becoming a sinking ship and I no longer wanted to be a part of it. This wasn't just the case with me, as the manager who had approached me not too long ago had also left for similar issues. When I felt I had enough of all I could take, I contacted her. She had left Baylor and went to UT Southwestern. Coincidentally, she happened to be working under Dr. Collins, who built the program there and whom I had interviewed with all those years earlier when first trying to break into this field. She told me about a position they had, which was basically the same position I had when I first started working at Baylor – data extracting and analysis for the submission to the national registry, CIBMTR. Things had gotten so bad where I was, I was actually considering this, even though I felt it would be a step back. I would go from the coordinating of patients under studies I managed, to working with databases. I was willing to do this though with the hopes of jumping into a Clinical Research Coordinator position when one became available at UT Southwestern. I had expressed my interest and I had an interview scheduled within a week.

During the interview, all I kept thinking was, am I really going to enjoy doing these forms again? Are things really this bad at Baylor? I was on the fence the whole time, back and forth, as I was being passed around from interviewer to interviewer. Then it was time to have my final interview, or so I thought. So far, I had met with the lady who would be my manger, as well as the person who served as the internal auditor. Both interviews went great and now I would be interviewing with Dr. Collins. I wondered if he'd remember me from the time he had interviewed me seven years later. Sure enough he did, and again, like he said last time we met, he again remarked, I should be the poster child for transplantation.

We began discussing what I had been up to since we last met and began talking about what I would like to be doing. We talked about various studies I had worked on at Baylor. We talked about the transplant study I had helped design and co-authored. We talked about some of the publications I had been in. We even talked about some studies I thought would be interesting to look at and manage. All in all, our interview took about an hour and a half, and as it was wrapping up, he asked if I could hold on a second while he checked something out and said he'd be right back. When he returned, he told me he felt I would be much more suited to be a Clinical Research Coordinator there at UT Southwestern, just as I had been at Baylor. I of course wholeheartedly agreed with his sentiments. He said he believed they were getting ready to open up a Clinical Research Coordinator position and had just checked on the status. The issue was at UT Southwestern, the Clinical Research Coordinators were all RN positions; however, I wasn't an RN – I thought here we go again. He felt with my experience and education, I was just as qualified, if not more so, than some of the RN's. He needed to see if an adjustment could be made to the position, opening it up to non-nurse candidates. He felt confident this would happen and he could help expedite the process if I was interested. He wanted me to next meet with the BMT/HemMalig research manager. Unfortunately, she wasn't there that day and I would have to come back again to meet with her.

Now that the interview was over and I was on my way back to Baylor, I was having difficulty in providing an excuse for why I was so late. I had initially told my manager I would be in late this morning arriving a little after 9:00 a.m., but here it was close to 1:00 p.m. I figured I would just play it by ear when and if anyone ever said anything and luckily, no one ever did. My manager had taken the day off and wasn't aware how late I had arrived, and I had no patients that morning, so no one was the wiser.

Later that week, I would return to UT Southwestern for the final interview with the research manager and all went well. I met the rest of the team, and felt confident all would work out. I was very excited at the prospect of working at UT Southwestern. They were NCI designated, were doing cutting edge research, and when I named the salary I was looking at and what it would take to pull me from Baylor, no one balked at it. I was stoked.

Meanwhile, as I waited for the final word from UT Southwestern, work at Baylor was feeling more and more like work and less like something I enjoyed. I was extremely eager for something to happen with UT Southwestern and sure enough, about three months after I interviewed, I received a call from HR extending an offer to me – I accepted.

I must admit it was bitter sweet leaving Baylor, as I had been there for seven years. It's where I got my start and obtained a great deal of knowledge in this field that had become so much more to me than just a job. It was enjoyable though to see the reaction on my manger's face when I handed in my letter of resignation and one month's notice. She definitely wasn't expecting I'd ever leave, which is probably why it was so easy to take advantage of me. No more though, not this time. I was out. I must admit, I was a little shocked they didn't even ask me to stay, but I take solace in the fact that the transplant physicians I had worked with for so long did make an attempt. However, they were told to back down by the administration.

My last day at Baylor, consisted of a 15-hour day, until around 10:00 p.m., when I finally just told myself, there was no way I was going to get everything done I needed to get done. I just needed to leave and let whomever was going to take my patients and studies, figure it out without me. It was time for me to begin a new chapter and I was excited for the opportunity UT Southwestern had given me.

Working at UT Southwestern was a bit unnerving. I was quickly learning during my first week, that although I had done the exact same thing at Baylor, UT Southwestern had a lot more processes and structure, and learning all these things took some time. Additionally, one of my new co-workers who happened to be training me only worked two days a week, which limited the ability for me to be trained, not to mention, she had also just learned she was pregnant and decided to hand in her two week's notice and be a stay-at-home mom. None of this really mattered though, as I was given studies and patients immediately. This worked out great and actually best for me as the best way for me to learn a new system is to be thrown in.

As I was getting settled in at UT Southwestern, IUI procedure number 2 was now upon us and again we were extremely excited and well prepared. With our first attempt, we felt one thing that could have gone awry was our miscalculating the ovulation peak. Just being off a day or two could have caused the procedure to misfire. To ensure this didn't happen again, we were going to 'trigger' the ovulation. This would allow us to exactly pinpoint when the peak was happening and sure enough, about a week and a half later, the home pregnancy test came back positive and we were elated. I couldn't believe this was really happening and there are no words to accurately describe our emotions.

The hardest thing about being pregnant at this point, was keeping the news to ourselves. We knew the golden rule as far as not telling anyone until we were in the clear so to speak – about three months down the line. We both agreed not to tell anyone until we reached this first milestone and we stuck to this for about eight weeks, when we could no longer keep it to ourselves. My grandparent's 55th anniversary was coming up, so we decided we would make them a picture book full of photos of us and Landon with the sonogram of our newest family member stuck somewhere in the middle. We handed the picture book to my grandparents and they were being grandparents, doting on us and how adorable Landon was and blessed we all were. Then all of the sudden we here, "What? What's that say – Hi Mom and Dad?," just as the sonographer typed it, and then my parents were like wait, what was that, and then the tears started flowing. It was a great way of breaking the news to them and a great memory as well. We finished our weekend celebration and then vowed not to tell anyone else until we had reached the next major milestone. Luckily work was keeping me busy and since I was new, I didn't really feel a need to share our news with anyone else at that point.

Things were great for all of us. Landon was thriving in his daycare, shocking us daily with all the new things he was learning. His vocabulary had exploded and was speaking in both English and Mandarin. We couldn't have been happier with how things were working out. I had been at UT Southwestern for several months now and getting used to how things worked there. I was learning how to navigate the system there. I was pleased with my decision to leave Baylor, as not only was my pay better, but my benefits were as well. My whole family was able to go on my insurance for just a little bit more than what we were paying for only me at Baylor. Additionally, I had a state-backed pension, which is really unheard of these days. Work was also going great. I was getting more and more patients and receiving more and more studies. My new team even gave Elisse and I a nice gift card for our newest addition coming soon.

Baby #2, son #2, that's right another son, was developing right on track with no issues whatsoever. We were kind of hoping for a girl, so we could have one of each, but I must admit, I was pretty okay with two boys – besides, I still had three more vials left, so a girl (perhaps another boy) was still a possibility.

We were about eight months along now and I say we, not because I was carrying the baby, but because I was just as involved as I could have been with the pregnancy at the time. I would get up in the middle of the night to get my wife whatever she needed. I went to every check-up with her. Consulted the same books, and didn't miss anything. I'd say I was definitely hands on. We went in for our week 36 visit on Friday and the doctor said the baby is measuring about six pounds and is tracking on schedule and should be around eight pounds at birth. I do believe it was apparent, the thought of an eight pound baby shooting out of my wife was a bit frightening to her, but I wasn't worried in the least bit and was ready. I just told her to relax, which helped and provided as much comfort as you would it expect it to.

The next day, Saturday, began a very busy and hectic weekend for us. We still needed to get some last-minute preparations set up for when the baby came. We didn't have our hospital bag ready. We didn't even have a name picked out yet, but were narrowing this down. We needed to decide want to do with Landon when it was time to go to the hospital. We needed to do a practice run, so we knew how much time it would take. We had time, but not a lot. We did at least feel we had thought of everything though at this point, but of course we missed one thing. We didn't think how or what we would do if our baby came early, and the very next day, none of it mattered anyway, because without warning baby # 2 was coming whether we were ready or not.

As Sunday rolled around, we were headed on our way out to the store to pick up some groceries, when our phone rang. It was one of my mom's friends from college, Marsha. She lived a few miles from us and had known me since I was born. Given all the preparations we still had to make, I told Elisse to just let it go to voicemail and we'd call her back when we got back from the store. Elisse felt compelled to answer though. Marsha wanted to bring over a gift for the soon to be arriving baby boy. I told Elisse she should have let it go to voicemail because now we we're going to be here at the house for a while waiting.

Now rarely in my life have I been wrong (Elisse can confirm this), but I sure was wrong that day, for if Marsha hadn't have come over that day, my wife's water would have broke in Wal-Mart, placing us, without a doubt on the evening news, birthing our son at the local Wal-Mart. When Marsha left, Elisse reached to put down the gift Marsha had brought us, and "POP." I heard my wife scream, which resulted in me running around the corner to see what was going on. She said she thought her water broke. I asked if she was sure, as we were just at the check-up Friday and everything was tracking on scheduled. How could we be 3.5 weeks early now?

Elisse called her doctor who told her to get to the hospital immediately, but at my wife's request the doctor agreed she could shower, as long as there were no contractions, otherwise we needed to get there immediately. My wife jumped in the shower, while I loaded the car. This didn't take any time at all, as we were 3.5 weeks early and didn't really have much to load. We called a friend to come watch Landon and we left. Elisse knew from our birth classes that once you get to the hospital, food was not an option until the baby came, so of course she begged me to swing in somewhere to get some food. I told her not a chance. I wasn't risking anything and went straight to the hospital. We got in and settled and by then the contractions were already two minutes apart.

My wife was a super trooper when it came to labor and I was extremely proud of her. I always knew she was tough, but I had no idea the threshold of pain she had. As the contractions became stronger and stronger, her time between the contractions became less and less to where she was pretty much having a constant contraction. We had gotten to the hospital about 3:30 p.m. and at 8:30 p,m., we we're far enough along that she wouldn't be able to receive Pitocin. This was our goal at this point, as we didn't want to run the risk of getting into a slippery slope of having to do a c-section if the Pitocin put the baby in distress. Since we were past the "Pitocin window," Elisse went ahead and requested an epidural. This greatly relieved her pain, slowed the contractions, and most of all, allowed Elisse to get some rest.

At this point my parents had arrived and we went to grab a bite to eat while Elisse rested. Not too much longer after we had finished eating, I had gotten back to the room and had a chance to try to get a little sleep. I laid my head on the pillow, and just as I closed my eyes, in walked the delivery team. It was time and we were ready to meet him and about two hours later, we did. Huxton had arrived, a healthy perfect baby boy who was fully developed only pre-term weighing in at 5 lbs. 9 oz. Elisse again reiterated how glad she was Huxton came early, as she couldn't have imagined delivering him at eight pounds. We stayed in the hospital for another two days and then we were off to home with our newest member of our family.

This period in our lives was definitely full of joy and lots of questions. From 18 months and on, we were good to go, but at this stage, newborn to 18 months was all new to us.

We consulted many books on SIDS, co-sleeping, when to call the doctor, when to relax, breast feeding vs. formula and many others. Landon, being Landon was also a blessing during this time. He was, and still is a wonderful big brother, very helpful and very excited to have a little brother. In fact, I remember the day we told, rather confirmed to him we were pregnant. He was overjoyed. For several weeks whenever he asked if mommy had a baby in her tummy, we would ask why he thought that and he would explain mommy's tummy was growing.

We didn't want him to get too excited in the beginning before we knew we were in the clear, and we hadn't really discussed what we were going to say. Being the persistent little boy he is, he kept pressing, so one day, I just blurted out mommy's been eating a lot more food lately. I'm not sure Elisse agreed with that approach, but as I said, we hadn't really talked about what we would say to Landon when pressed. In any case, when it did come time to tell him, when we asked if he remembered wondering why mommy's tummy was growing, he just started jumping up and down exclaiming, "...I'm gonna have a little brother, I'm gonna have a little brother...." He was so excited and we were so excited we had a son so we didn't have to burst his bubble and tell him he was having a little sister instead.

We were so fortunate to have such a blessing and we were truly amazed then, and now, at how Huxton had been on ice for 12 years prior – truly a miraculous event.

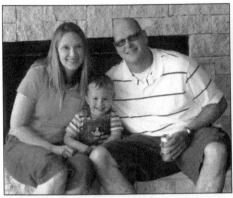

Elisse, Landon, and I at my parent's house in Lago Vista before the adoption was final. Landon is 2 at this time and I'm about 8 years post transplant.

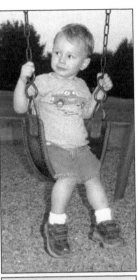

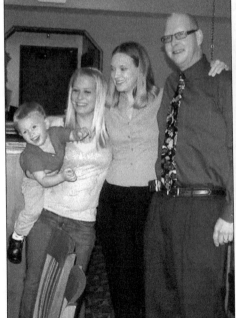

Landon, his birth-mother (Jordy), Elisse and myself – Adoption finalized

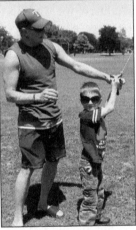

"Dad and son" spending quality time together flying a kite

⊔ SOUTHWESTERN
MEDICAL CENTER

Daniel K. Podolsky, M.D.
President
Philip O'Bryan Montgomery, Jr., M.D. Distinguished
Presidential Chair in Academic Administration

Professor of Internal Medicine
Doris and Bryan Wildenthal Distinguished
Chair in Medical Science

Welcome to UT Southwestern Medical Center

I would like to be one of the first to welcome you to UT Southwestern Medical Center, a world-class medical institution and employer of choice in North Texas. UT Southwestern exemplifies what an academic medical institution can and should be—a diverse community of exceptionally talented people who are committed to achieving our goal of a top performing academic health care system.

Our faculty includes many who are the top scholars in their fields. They are actively engaged in teaching, research, and patient care. The staff that work alongside them are equally skilled and passionate, and as you will very soon discover, are the strength upon which our success has been built. I am delighted that you have decided to join them in our collective mission to:

- improve health care in our community, Texas, our nation, and the world through innovation;
- educate the next generation of leaders in patient care, biomedical science, and disease prevention;
- conduct high-impact, internationally recognized biomedical research; and
- deliver patient care that brings UT Southwestern's scientific advances to the bedside—focusing on quality, safety, and service.

I again welcome you to UT Southwestern Medical Center. I hope your employment with us is filled with growth, satisfaction, and discovery.

Sincerely,

Daniel K. Podolsky, M.D.

5323 Harry Hines Blvd. / Dallas, Texas 75390-9002 / 214-648-2508   Fax 214-648-8690
www.utsouthwestern.edu

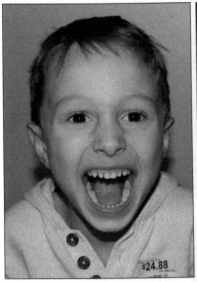

Landon at about 4 years old and soon to be a big brother

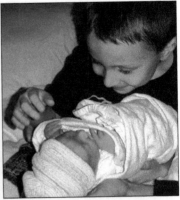

Excitement abounds!

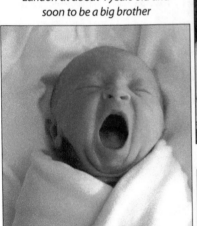

After being on ice for 12 years and thanks to the miracle of child birth, science, God, and IUI, our newest addition (Huxton) arrives. He's 2 days old here and very tired.

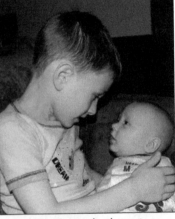

Figuring each other out

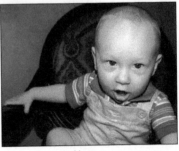

Huxton

CHAPTER 10: NEW LIFE

It's crazy to think of the path my life has taken over the past two decades. When this crazy journey started, I was on top of the world getting ready to start my new life with my soon to be wife and working in my new job and living in our new house. Elisse and I had our whole futures ahead of us, and then in the blink of an eye, everything changed. Never once did I wonder why me or what have I done to deserve this, but at times, while going through the treatment especially, I did often times wonder how long would it take for things to get back to normal, if ever. When were there going to be more good days than bad ones? The search for normalcy is a challenging one, and when I was first diagnosed with leukemia, I wasn't sure what to expect or what would happen. The certainty of uncertainty was the only thing I was certain of.

Often times I sit back and wonder what my life would have been like had I never been diagnosed with leukemia now 17 years ago. Let me count the ways. First and foremost, we wouldn't have been fortunate enough to have Landon, one of the most precious things, gifts, in our lives. If Elisse and I were able to have babies the normal way, as if I had never gone through chemo and radiation which resulted in my sterility, we would have had no reason to explore adoption in the first place. Much in the same manner, for the same reasons, we wouldn't have had the equally other precious gift we have been so blessed with – Huxton, now four years old. There would have been no reason 17 years ago, to sperm bank. Regarding my choice of employment, I truly believe it chose me. Had I not gone through this journey, most likely I would have continued working in the telecom field. Who knows, perhaps I could have developed Facebook, rather than Zuckerberg. Perhaps Elisse might not have been a lawyer. Instead of waiting nine years to have children, we probably would have had them two or three years after we were married, and law school with children is an almost impossibility, although I'm sure if anyone could've done it, it would be Elisse. From early on, Elisse and I had been through the hardest, most difficult times most couples will never have to go through, ever; and this has provided a foundation that can surely handle anything that attempts to shake it.

I would have had to move from my apartment to our first house, but instead, I was in the hospital undergoing chemo – everybody hates to move. I went on the fastest most effective diet out there, although, I don't recommend it to anyone, but I lost 70 lbs. in four months and although I am now a healthier 215 lbs., I have a super high metabolism that doesn't seem to allow me to get over 220 lbs. no matter how hard I try. Again I don't recommend this diet, but it was very effective.

Excellent health care by a variety of specialists, as when one goes through transplant, they are instantaneously thrown into a world of medical specialists from all areas of medicine and "waiting" to get in to see one is something that never happens. Same day service is the rule, not the exception.

Elisse and I always have a large cushion in place, a nest egg if you will, because as we learned the hard way that you never know when your life will be turned upside down.

These are just the ways I can count up to this point in my life, but as I've learned through this journey, there will be countless more that I can't even imagine. The unique gift of perspective is probably the most grounding one I've received in all this. I have learned that no matter how bad I think I have it, there is always someone out there who would kill to have the troubles I have had.

Yes, I have stared death in the face and lived to tell about it, but often that is not the case. I often think of the three year old – Taylor – who was going through her second transplant, especially now as I look at my own children. I couldn't imagine how, if even possible, I would get through the ordeal of having a child go through chemo, radiation, transplantation and eventually having to say an earthly goodbye.

Since the time I was diagnosed and started working in clinical research, there have been upwards of 70 patients I have personally come in contact with, either by a clinical trial they were on that I coordinated, or through a LLS First Connections, or just friends of friends, that weren't as fortunate as I was. The flip side to this, of course, is there are countless more out there that have made it, and that is the most rewarding fulfilling aspect I have been fortunate to enough to experience through working in the field that saved my life.

People often asked me how hard transplantation was and I can honestly say it was by far, without a doubt, the hardest thing I have ever had to go through, but being almost 17 years out now, it's a very surreal feeling. I know I went through it, but it also seems as if it was someone else that went through it, which seems strange I know. I can't explain it to others except to say hopefully you'll never go through something like that, but you will understand if you do.

My life now is as normal as any persons at this point – I go to my oncologist annually just for a blood test – pretty routine.

Landon and Huxton are best buds and get along far better than my sister and I ever did. I'm told this will change, but still enjoying it now. Elisse has since left the firm she worked at and has started her own firm and is enjoying all the freedom that provides. I look back on the path my life has taken me and I wouldn't change any of it. What started out as something full of uncertainty, fear, and potential death, resulted in a life far better than I ever could have imagined for myself, and thankfully I, no we, our family, have plenty more life to live.

The future is something I never really worry about, because I know it will get here day by day and when I'm old looking back at my life, who really knows what other amazing things I will have as memories to hold onto. It is truly a blessing to have gone through what I have gone through and I strongly believe none of the things that truly bring me joy today would be here if I hadn't been fortunate enough to have had my world turned upside down by that frightening diagnosis of leukemia that seemed like a lifetime ago.

I truly owe my life to my sister for without her life saving bone marrow, I wouldn't be here today writing this book, or enjoying my life. Of course, I owe my live to the doctors as well, and to the nurses who really are the nuts and bolts of medicine. Elisse of course, was here in my life with me before my diagnosis, but stayed with me and helped battle this disease which ending up being a gift in disguise. My parents provided continued unwavering support. And finally, I owe my life to the one who made all this possible, for which without, none of this would have happened – God.

There are also constant reminders of this journey – this path I was placed on, especially with my kids and all the other reminders listed above. In addition to those, there are also health-related reminders that keep me on my toes, risks of secondary malignancies, long-term latent effects of radiation and chemo – organ damage. These constant possibilities always reside in the midbrain. I say midbrain, because I refuse to worry about things I cannot control. However, I'm not so caviler about them that they reside in the background either.

I've been conditioned to recognize it's much easier to control and manage anything better the earlier it's picked up, before they become too large to control or manage. I'm 41 years old now and already have cataracts starting to form. My cholesterol as of late is something that has started to rise. There is an increased risk of skin cancer post-transplant, and with me, the risk is 100% increased, as I have already had three areas of basal cell carcinoma removed. I've had more colonoscopies now, than the average person has by the time they turn 60. In fact, I'm due for my fifth one shortly, and each one has demonstrated polyps with one being precancerous. All these things would be considered burdensome to most people I believe, but for me and what I've been through, I welcome these minor inconveniences in life, as I am just happy I am around to need to have them.

I'm not sure who will read this book, if it will ever be published, and if anyone will ever read it. The main purpose for this book is to capture my story, so when I'm old, gray, and forgetful, I will have a record of what happened all those years earlier, as will my kids. It is also my hope that perhaps other people diagnosed with a cancer of some sort, or their family member, will find some sort of solace or comfort in knowing that people can make it through. No matter how bad things may seem presently, in the end it may lead to something completely unexpected.

The future remains bright and I'm extremely optimistic and excited to see what it has in store for me, but it truly remains unwritten at this point and is why this chapter is so short.

I look forward to participating in this story called life and perhaps there will be a part two of this story someday, but for right now, I'm glad and overly thankful to have made it this far and look forward to all the twist, turns, and curve balls life throws my way.

Note that a percentage of all book sales will be donated to the Leukemia and Lymphoma Society.

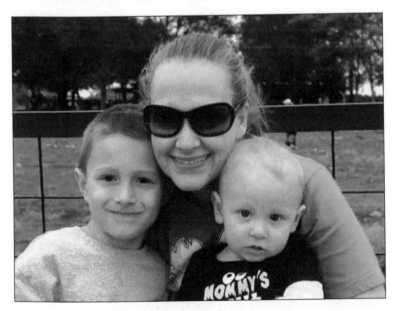

Mom and her boys

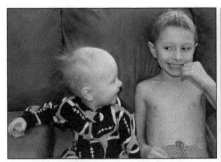

Huxton and Landon – Best buds

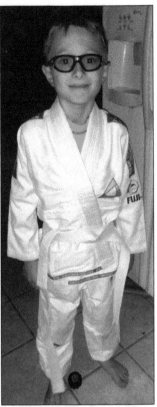

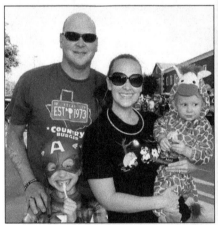

Halloween. I'm about 13 years
post transplant

Landon ready for jujitsu

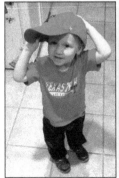

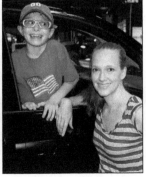

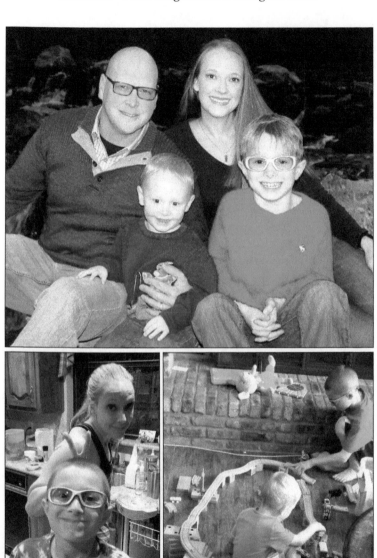

Brothers building trains

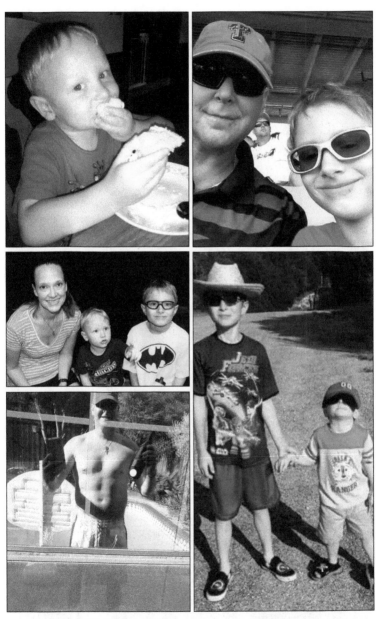

Gaining weight – enjoying life!   *Best buds*

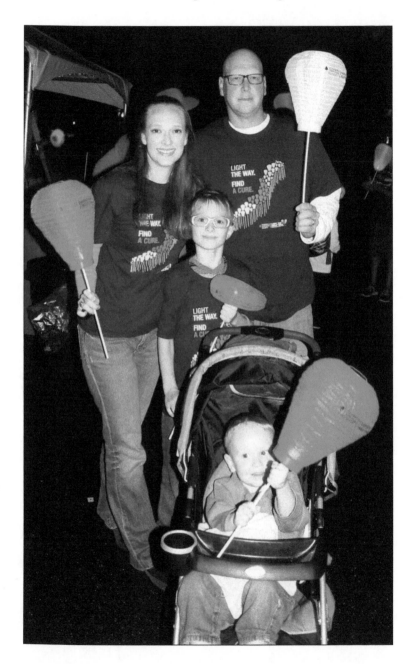

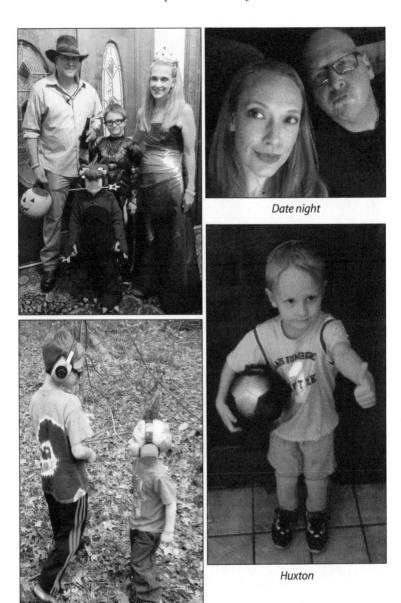

Date night

Huxton

Landon and Huxton

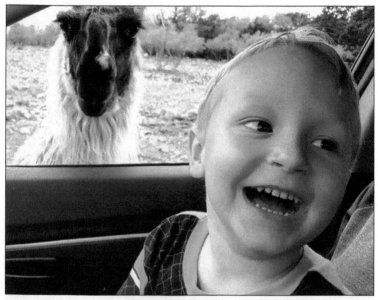

Wildlife reserve

Family at the circus. I'm about 16 years post transplant

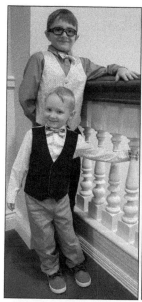

Easter

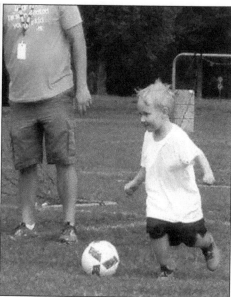

Huxton playing soccer

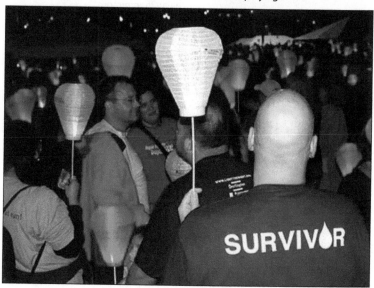

Still surviving at 17+ years post transplant

LIST OF RESOURCES

American Cancer Society –
Hotel Partners Program
1-800-227-2345

Be The Match
www.bethematch.org
1-800-627-7692

Cancer Care
www.cancercare.org
1-800-813-4673

Cancer Legal Resource Center
www.cancerlegalresources.org
1-866-843-2572

Cancer Support Community
www.cancersupportcommunity.org
1-888-793-9355

Good Days
www.mygooddays.org
1-877-963-7233

Heroes For Children
www.heroesforchildren.org

Imerman Angels
www.imermanangels.org
1-866-463-7626

Leukemia and Lymphoma Society
www.lls.org
1-800-955-4572

Leukemia Texas
www.leukemiatexas.org

Multiple Myeloma Research Foundation
www.themmrf.org

Patient Advocate Foundation
www.patientadvocate.org
1-800-532-5274

Triage Cancer
www.triagecancer.org